Instructor's Manual
and Test Bank

for

D1450767

Bishop and Aldana
Step Up to Wellness
A Stage-Based Approach

prepared by

Jan Galen Bishop
Richard Bishop

Allyn and Bacon
Boston   London   Toronto   Sydney   Tokyo   Singapore

Table of Contents

Test Bank

Preface

This instructor's manual and test bank was written to help instructors prepare for and teach wellness concepts using the text, *Step Up to Wellness: A Stage-Based Approach*. In this book you will find a summary, objectives, personal profiles, a content outline, behavior boosts, additional student activities, lab exercises, behavior change information, and a list of resources. Included are suggested readings, a list of professional organizations, video and film selections, and additional local and community resources for each of the 15 chapters presented in the textbook.

The summary was included to provide instructors with a brief overview of what students should learn from each chapter. This is detailed in the objectives which are listed. Each chapter of this instructor's manual also includes a personal profile. These profiles are true stories of how noted Americans were able to adopt different aspects of a wellness lifestyle. They are intended to show how famous actors, politicians, and professionals were able to make lifestyle changes part of everyday living. Hopefully, students will hear these and realize that they are not alone in their efforts to reduce health risk.

The most important part of this manual is the detailed outlines which describe the content of each chapter. Great efforts were taken to assure that each chapter outline contained as much detail as possible. By following the outlines, you should be able to address each and every item of each chapter.

Each chapter also contains behavior boosts which are short verbal tips on how to change poor behaviors or maintain good ones. They are followed by additional student assessments and lab exercises and additional stages of change information. We hope each of these items will assist you in reaching your students. References to other books or related articles have been included, as well as a list of videos and professional organizations which can help you teach these concepts more effectively.

Finally, there are over 825 carefully written test questions which can be used to evaluate the cognitive portion of your classes. These questions include multiple choice, true/false, and essay questions, with the correct responses directly below the questions. Following the correct responses for multiple choice questions is a number shown in parentheses. This number ranges from one to three and is a measure of the difficulty of the question. Questions marked with a one are the easiest and tend to be factual. Questions marked with a three are the most difficult. Mix and match questions of varying difficulty as you prepare your exams. We hope this manual will simplify your teaching assignments and help your students step up to wellness.

Discovering the Wellness Lifestyle

Chapter 1

CHAPTER SUMMARY

Wellness is a way of life. It means taking responsibility for one's own health and well-being and adopting lifestyle habits that maximize quality of life and minimize risk of disease and premature death. Personal wellness can be broken down into five dimensions: physical, mental, emotional, social, and spiritual wellness. Each of these dimensions shares equally in a person's well being and each dimension interacts with the other four. Striving for wellness usually means making changes, replacing negative lifestyle behaviors with positive ones. Change can be difficult and not everyone is equally ready to embark on change, let alone on the same changes. For that reason, the Stages of Change Model is presented in this chapter. This model recognizes individual differences in readiness to change and explains how to use stage-appropriate strategies to move through behavior change. Through stages of change, everyone can achieve a greater level of wellness.

LEARNING OBJECTIVES

The students will be able to:
- define quality of life.
- explain the relationship between quality of life and personal lifestyle habits.
- identify unhealthy personal lifestyle habits and target one or two for change.
- define, compare, and contrast the concepts of health and wellness.
- define quality of life and explain how it can be affected by a wellness lifestyle.
- describe the illness to wellness continuum.
- describe the five dimensions of wellness.
- identify the impact of lifestyle habits on each dimension of wellness.
- list and explain the four factors responsible for all causes of death.
- describe and characterize the five stages of the behavior change model.
- identify personal lifestyle habits that, if changed, would result in a better quality of life

PERSONAL PROFILE

Change Your Future Today

At age 23, Victoria Santos reached an important milestone—she graduated from college. "It wasn't always easy and sometimes I thought that maybe I just wasn't capable of getting a degree. In the beginning some of my classes were so overwhelming that I felt lost and confused, but when I look back now, they don't seem so difficult. Education has helped me better understand myself, other people and the world around me. Not only am I qualified for a good job, I'm also a more mature person than when I started college."

Victoria's education has prepared her to make the important decisions that face almost all adults between the ages of 18 and 30. Some of these decisions include: What should I do for the rest of my life? What jobs do I apply for? Whom should I date or marry? What about children? How will I pay for my school loans? In addition, other decisions that may seem less important can have a cumulative effect on the quality of life and overall happiness. Decisions like: What shall I have for dinner? Should I exercise regularly? If I drink alcohol, how much can I safely consume?

The knowledge Victoria gained in college has altered many aspects of her life. During her first years, the demands of school, work, and dating seemed to occupy all of her time, and regular exercise had never been a part of her life. "I was never very good at sports and did not particularly enjoy exercise," she said. "Every time I went hiking, jogging, or did anything vigorous, I felt tired and out of breath. It was also hard to be involved in exercise when I had a few extra pounds that the others didn't have. To save myself from discomfort and embarrassment, I just didn't make time for exercise." But some of Victoria's friends who exercised often encouraged her to work out with them. Their encouragement and example helped her discover that exercise did not have to be painful, embarrassing, or difficult. To them, exercise was fun. "As I slowly overcame the barriers that kept me from exercising, both my attitude and body weight gradually changed. I knew I'd have to improve my diet, too, to make the whole thing work, so I took a nutrition class as one of my electives and then followed up with one of the nutrition counselors on campus. I feel better about myself and I feel better physically, too. I'm still as busy as ever, but now I know that the time I spend exercising is a wise investment in me and my future. I know I'm not perfect, but now I have confidence in my ability to learn and keep improving." With a degree in hand, a willingness to learn and change, and a lifestyle full of healthy habits, Victoria has every reason to be optimistic about her future.

CONTENT OUTLINE

I. Healthy behaviors increase the likelihood of living longer with less disease.
    A. People who exercise regularly will, on the average, live longer than those who don't.
    B. People who don't use tobacco have a lower risk for cancer and heart disease.
II. Striving for wellness often requires a person to change lifestyle behaviors.
    A. Change can be difficult.
    B. Change requires readiness, commitment, and resources.
    C. Not everyone is equally ready to make lifestyle changes.
    D. A person can be in different stages of readiness for different lifestyle behaviors.
    E. Readiness to change is influenced by many factors including:
        1. personality
        2. living and work environments
        3. family support
III. The concept of wellness has evolved from a holistic point of view that sees the human individual as a complex interdependent mixture of physical, emotional, social, mental and spiritual factors.
    A. Each of these five factors, or dimensions, of wellness is equally important.

B. Personal choice influences:
1. one's own wellness
2. the wellness of people with whom we interact
3. the wellness of the world in which we live

IV. Wellness means striving for quality living.
A. A high quality of life means feeling good about oneself and being able to do most of the things you want to do despite any limitations you may have.
B. A low quality of life is characterized by a dependence on others for basic needs, having a poor self-concept, being too ill to effectively communicate or take part in a relationship, or being unable to do the things you want to do.
1. while illnesses or disabilities can negatively affect quality of life, they need not deter one from living a wellness lifestyle and achieving personal potential
C. The average life span has increased but the ratio of healthy to dysfunctional years hasn't changed much since 1995 when it was 63.7 years of healthy (quality) living and 12.1 years of dysfunctional (poor quality) living.
1. a wellness lifestyle can reduce the number of dysfunctional years and may also increase life span
2. no one has complete control over health and life—a wellness lifestyle limits the risk of disease and accidents; it doesn't ensure total health
3. life span has increased from 47 years in 1900 to 75.8 years in 1995
4. major reasons for an increasing life span by era:
a. Age of Environment (1900–1936): reduction in illness and disease, city and federal health campaigns, medical discoveries (e.g. insulin), public health measures like pasteurization of milk
b. Age of Medicine (1937–1949): ability to cure some diseases, dramatic changes in medicine occurred with the discovery of bacteria-killing drugs (antibiotics and penicillin)
c. Age of Lifestyle (1950–1989): majority of premature deaths resulted from poor lifestyle habits; 75% were preventable by 1989, medical advances like heart transplants did not increase the average life span, good lifestyle habits did
d. Age of Wellness (1990–): small increments in life span, additional gains will likely be the result of further lifestyle changes and new knowledge of the human body

V. Wellness means being proactive.
A. Many people are content to be in the middle of the illness-to-wellness continuum.
1. symptom-free people often ignore warnings of lifestyle risk
2. rather than practice prevention, many people depend on medicine to fix them
B. The wellness movement is characterized by taking personal control of one's own wellness and striving not just for the absence of disease but for a quality of life that encompasses physical, emotional, mental, spiritual and social health.
1. the World Health Organization expanded its definition of health to "a state of complete physical, mental, and social well-being and not merely the absence of disease."
2. a proactive stance means actively :

        a.   participating in regular physical activity

        b.   controlling stress

        c.   eating a proper diet

        d.   practicing cancer and cardiovascular disease prevention

        e.   managing body weight

        f.   avoiding harmful substances and infectious diseases

        g.   enjoying healthy relationships

        h.   encouraging spiritual development

        i.   caring for the environment

VI.   The five dimensions of wellness are physical, spiritual, emotional, social, and mental health.

    A.   Physical Dimension

        1.   participation in regular physical activity

            a.   health experts believe that large improvements in national health could be realized if the sedentary portion of the population were to adopt physically active lifestyles

                (1)   sixty percent of adults do not exercise regularly.

                (2)   people with poor fitness levels have 8 times higher risk of death due to cardiovascular disease and 5 times higher probability of dying from cancer than persons who have good or excellent levels of fitness

            b.   some physical activities are health-related, others more skill-related.

                (1)   the five health-related components of physical fitness are:

                    (a)   cardiorespiratory endurance (fitness)

                    (b)   joint flexibility

                    (c)   muscular strength

                    (d)   muscular endurance

                    (e)   body composition

                (2)   benefits of regular physical activity include (see also chapter two):

                    (a)   increased endurance and less fatigue

                    (b)   weight loss, decreased risk of diabetes

                    (c)   decreased risk of diseases, e.g. cancer, heart disease, osteoporosis

                    (d)   increased immune response

                    (e)   psychological benefits, e.g. decreased depression, stress, etc.

        2.   managing stress

        3.   preventing alcohol and substance abuse

        4.   avoiding sexually transmitted diseases

    B.   Spiritual Dimension

        1.   coming to peace with one's self and discovering a sense of purpose

        2.   believing in and adhering to personal morals and values

        3.   viewing present events and misfortunes in a long-range perspective

        4.   the role of religion as a component of spiritual wellness

    C.   Emotional Dimension

        1.   the ability to handle emotions in a constructive way resulting in a positive emotional state

        2.   happiness stems from the ability to love oneself and others, and feel loved in return

3. the personality trait of hostility is a predictor of heart attacks
4. a positive attitude, sometimes referred to as a hardiness, promotes health and wellness
5. laughter at oneself is a sign of emotional balance

    D. Social Dimension
1. the ability to have positive interactions with others including friends, family, work-related personnel
2. loving relationships promote physical and mental health
3. "nice" people tend to have a higher quality of life

    E. Mental Dimension
1. the ability to continually learn, think clearly, make good decisions, and adapt to new circumstances
2. the ability to be creative and imaginative
3. knowledge is a powerful tool in preventing illness and disease
4. viewing difficult situations as challenges and opportunities for growth

VII. Factors influencing wellness
    A. Heredity
    B. Environment
    C. Inadequate health care
    D. Lifestyle

VIII. Reaching wellness through lifestyle change
    A. Awareness
1. to make change, a person must be aware of, and buy into the need to change
2. to make change, a person must be able to distinguish between good and bad lifestyle behaviors

    B. Assessment
1. heightens awareness.
2. helps determine how much change (if any) is needed.
3. establishes a baseline from which change can be measured (See Lab 1.1)

IX. Stages of Change Model (Transtheoretical Model of Change)
    A. My behavior change programs have low success rates
1. only 5 % of dieters are able to reach and maintain an optimal body weight after 2 years.
2. most smokers have to quit a number of times before they succeed

    B. Drs. James Prochaska and Carlo DiClemente and colleagues studied how people change and proposed the Stages of Change Model. The model is based on the belief that people are in different stages of readiness to change and that the processes of change (strategies) must match the stage of readiness. The five stages are:
1. Precontemplators: are not thinking about changing their behavior
2. Contemplators: are seriously thinking about making change
3. Preparers: have made the decision to change a behavior but have not taken consistent action to change it
4. Action Takers: have made the change and are consistently practicing the new behavior but have only been doing so for 6 months or less
5. Maintainers: are committed to a behavior and have maintained it for 6 months or more

C.   A person can be in different stages for different health behaviors.

D.   Movement can occur linearly between stages or jump stages. One can also fall back and then jump ahead again.

E.   Behavior change strategies (processes of change) are more effective when they are stage-based. (The following lists are a little simplistic—some strategies will work in several stages. For example awareness plays a role in the first 2–3 stages but is less important in the latter stages.)

    1.   moving from precontemplator to contemplator
        a.   awareness activities: information gathering, assessments, introspection
        b.   identification of supports and barriers
        c.   weighing of pros and cons

    2.   moving from contemplation to preparation
        a.   continued information gathering
        b.   continued weighing of pros and cons, pros being emphasized
        c.   goal setting, writing a contract

    3.   moving from preparation to action taker
        a.   develop a plan of action based on goals
        b.   remove triggers (barriers) and use supports
        c.   have a plan in the event of relapse
        d.   measure progress and evaluate goals

    4.   moving from action taker to maintainer
        a.   have a plan in the event of relapse
        b.   have plans to prevent relapse
        c.   find, create and use sources of motivation and support

BEHAVIOR BOOSTS

None for this introductory chapter.

SUGGESTED STUDENT ACTIVITIES

Activity 1: Lifestyle Habits: The Good and the Bad

Identify some of your "good" and "bad" lifestyle habits. Now rank the "bad" lifestyles with the one you feel most ready to change at the top, and the one you don't want to change or feel the least ready to tackle at the bottom.

Activity 2: Ten Ways to Enhance Your Wellness

Personal health behaviors and habits can play a major role in the quality of our lives. Here are ten ways you can enhance your wellness. Mark the ones that you think you currently practice. Then add any additional ideas you have for improving wellness.

1. Exercise regularly.

2. Maintain a safe level of blood cholesterol.
3. Control excessive body fat.
4. Eat a low-fat diet.
5. Develop successful relationships/interact well with others.
6. Get the necessary amount of sleep.
7. Avoid substance abuse, including tobacco.
8. Avoid alcohol or use it only in moderation.
9. Wear a seatbelt.
10. Gain happiness by doing for others.

Activity 3: What are Your Risks?

Take a moment to compile a list of things under the following two headings.

1. Things that you do that put you at more risk for accidents, illness, or death.
2. Things that you do that lower your risk and therefore enhance the quality of your life and perhaps extend it as well.

If you are comfortable doing so, share some of your actions, habits, and behaviors with a friend or small group of classmates.

LABS

1.1 Health and Wellness Inventory, p. 19–21
1.2 Healthy Lifestyle Evaluation, p. 22
1.3 Behavior Change Contract p. 23–24

RESOURCES

Suggested Reading

American College of Sports Medicine. The recommended quantity and quality of exercise for developing and maintaining cardiorespiratory and muscular fitness in healthy adults. *Medicine and Science in Sports* 22(2):265-274, 1990.

Fletcher, G.F., et al. American Heart Association: Statement on exercise. *Circulation* 862726, 1992.

International Society of Sport Psychology. *Physical activity and psychological benefits*: Position statement 20:179, 1992.

Paffenbarger, R.S., Jr., R.T. Hyde, A.L. Wing, and C.C. Hsieh. Physical activity, all-cause mortality, and longevity of college alumni. *New England Journal of Medicine* 314:605-613, 1986.

8

Pate, R.R., et al. Physical activity and public health: A recommendation from the Centers for Disease Control and Prevention and the American College of Sports Medicine. *Journal of the American Medical Association* 273(5):402-407, 1995.

U.S. Department of Health and Human Services. *Physical activity and health: A report of the Surgeon General.* Centers for Disease Control and Prevention, National Centers for Chronic Disease Prevention and Health Promotion. Atlanta: The President's Council on Physical Fitness and Sports, 1996.

U.S. Department of Health and Human Services. *Healthy people 2000*: National health promotion and disease prevention objectives. DHHS Publication No (PHS) 91-50213. Washington, D.C.: U.S. Government Printing Office, 1990.

Prochaska, J.O., DiClemente, C. 1986. Toward a comprehensive model of change. In *Treating addictive behaviors*, edited by W. Miller and N. Healther. New York: Plenum.

Organizations

American Alliance of Health, Physical Education,
Recreation and Dance (AAHPERD)
1900 Association Drive
Reston, VA 20191-1599
Tel (800) 213-7193
E-mail: info@aahperd.org
Web site: http://www.aahperd.org

American College of Sports Medicine (ACSM)
P.O. Box 1440
Indianapolis, IN 46206-1440
Tel (317) 637-9200
Fax (317) 634-7817
Web site: http://www.acsm.org

American College of Surgeons
633 North Saint Clair Street
Chicago, IL 60611-3211
Tel (312) 202-5000 ·
Fax (312) 202-5001
Web site: http://www.facs.org

The American Dietetic Association
216 West Jackson Boulevard
Chicago, IL 60606-6995
Tel (312) 899-0040
Fax (312) 899-1979
Web site: http://www.eatright.org

American Heart Association
National Center
7272 Greenville Avenue
Dallas, TX 75231
Tel (800) AHA-USA1 (Customer Heart & Stroke Information)
Tel (888) MY-HEART (Women's Health Information)
Web site: http://www.aha.org

Cooper Institute for Aerobic Research (CIAR)
12330 Preston Road
Dallas, TX 75230
Tel (800) 635-7050
Fax (972) 341-3224
Web site: http://www.cooperinst.org

U.S. Department of Agriculture
14th & Independence Avenue SW
Washington, DC 20250
Tel (202) 720-2791
Web site: http://www.usda.gov

Food and Nutrition Information Center
Web site: http://www.nalusda.gov/fnic

American Medical Athletic Association (AMAA)

4405 East West Highway
Suite 405
Bethesda, MD 20804
Tel: (800) 776-2732
Web site: http://www.arfa.org/amaa

President's Council on Physical Fitness and Sports
(PCPFS)
450 Fifth Street, NW, Suite 7103
Washington, DC 20001
(202) 272-2451
Web site: http://www.hhs.gov/progorg/ophs/pcpfs

Additional Local and Community Resources

American Heart Association
Blue Cross/Blue Shield
County Recreation Departments
Governor's Council on Health and Fitness
State and County Health Departments

The Fitness Wellness Connection

Chapter 2

CHAPTER SUMMARY

Physical activity is a powerful change agent. It can have a positive effect on a wide variety of health-related issues such as body fat, cholesterol, blood pressure, self-concept, stress relief, and more. Substantial health benefits (as much as 80 percent) can be achieved by performing moderately intense activity for 30 minutes on most days. Greater health benefits and physical fitness are achieved when you perform more vigorous activities. The components of physical fitness that most directly impact health are cardiorespiratory fitness, muscular strength and endurance, flexibility, and body composition. Skill development is not as directly related to health, but being skilled makes sports activities more enjoyable, which in turn provides motivation to be active—the key to physical wellness.

LEARNING OBJECTIVES

The student will be able to:

·   discuss the benefits of physical activity on each of the five wellness dimensions.
·   explain how an expanded knowledge base in physical fitness and exercise has changed our perception of what types of activities are important to health and wellness.
·   name and define the five health-related components of physical fitness.
·   explain the importance of both health-related and skill-related components of physical fitness.
·   organize and list by bodily system the physical benefits of exercise.
·   define physical activity, exercise, and physical fitness.
·   use the components and principles of physical activity to design a physical activity session using an activity of your choice.

PERSONAL PROFILE

President George Bush

The most common reason people cite for not exercising is lack of time. With all the duties and responsibilities that come with the job of president of the United States, lack of time would certainly be a valid excuse. But, when President George Bush occupied the Oval Office, he demonstrated that the busiest executive in the world could make regular exercise a part of his demanding schedule. He made exercise a priority, and it became part of his daily routine. Most recent presidents and first ladies have done the same.

For former President Bush, exercise is an opportunity to refresh and invigorate his mental and physical well-being. His exercise schedule consists of daily exercise sessions of at least fifteen to twenty minutes. He likes to run for three or four miles or, if he walks, he goes at such a fast pace that most of his security personnel have difficulty keeping up. During these "power walks" he usually covers between five and six miles at a pace that is more like jogging for most people.

According to Burton Lee III, President Bush's personal physician, "the guy is in good shape, darn good shape." Bush's exercise program consists of a variety of activities. He has been known to play tennis with professional tennis stars as well as foreign dignitaries. He also enjoys lifting weights, doing the Stairmaster, and bicycling. He likes to golf, but doesn't very often because he'd rather work up a sweat when he exercises.

Most important, President Bush enjoys a high-quality life because he is in excellent physical condition. He is an example of how one can maintain a lifelong routine of regular physical activity despite a busy schedule.

Griffin, Glen. President Bush: He's busy, but he still makes time for exercise. The Physician and Sportmedicine, 18:(7)95-99, 1990.

CONTENT OUTLINE

VIII.   Activewear and Active Lifestyles
     A.   Even though at some point during the day American adults are dressed in activewear, more than 60 percent do not achieve the recommended amount of regular physical activity.
         1.   25 percent are not active at all
     B.   Physical inactivity is now considered to be as important a risk factor in CHD disease as smoking, high blood cholesterol and high blood pressure.
         1.   inactivity is presently more common among
             a.   women than men
             b.   African-Americans
             c.   Hispanic than white adults
             d.   older than younger people
             e.   less affluent people
             f.   more educated than less educated adults
     C.   Until the 1960s, exercise was primarily thought of as calisthenics, military training and sports play.
     D.   In 1968 Dr. Kenneth Cooper introduced the idea of aerobic exercise and revolutionized people's thinking about exercise and health.
         1.   created the noun "aerobics," which he defined as any sustained rhythmic large-muscle activity
         2.   his first book made people aware of the health benefits of aerobic activity
         3.   motivated many men and women to jog, swim, etc., for their health
     E.   In the 1970s tennis and racquet ball became the "boom" sports.
         1.   by the late 1970s, Jackie Sorenson had introduced aerobic dance, the "boom" activity of the 1980s

2.   during the 1970s, university professors began to specialize in exercise research

F.   In the 1980s the idea of combining fitness and health emerged

     1.   the medical community began to shift it emphasis for "fix" to "prevent" and health and fitness professionals started teaming up to share their wealth of combined knowledge

     2.   "Fit for Life" movement began on many college and university campuses

II.   Physical activity, exercise, and physical fitness

A.   Physical activity, exercise and physical fitness are closely related but not synonymous.

     1.   physical activity is the broadest term, and it can be defined as "any bodily movement produced by skeletal muscles that results in energy expenditure"

     2.   exercise is generally thought of as a planned event, a structured workout that will make you more physically fit

     3.   physical fitness describes what you become, a set of attributes you obtain, attributes that allow you to perform physical activities

III.   Health-related fitness versus skill-related fitness

A.   Until the early 1980s, the emphasis was on sport skills and performance, which was believed to be health promoting.

     1.   skill-related components of physical fitness

         a.   agility

         b.   balance

         c.   coordination

         d.   power

         e.   reaction time

         f.   speed

     2.   fitness tests involved skill-based activities like the softball throw and shuttle run

         a.   only students scoring in the top 15 percent received recognition

B.   In 1980 AAHPERD published a booklet describing two categories of physical fitness—health and skill-related fitness.

     1.   health-related components of physical fitness

         a.   cardiorespiratory endurance

         b.   body composition

         c.   flexibility

         d.   muscular endurance

         e.   muscular strength

     2.   in 1984 AAHPERD published a set of health-related fitness tests

     3.   health-related tests include the one-mile run, sit-and-reach flexibility, and sit-ups

     4.   team sport curricula were modified to include lifetime activities such as tennis, golf, and archery

C.   Training for competition is different from exercising for health.

     1.   train long hours at high intensities

     2.   place your body in mechanically difficult positions

     3.   the motivation for intense practices and high-level performances comes from a deep-seated drive to excel and a desire to win recognition and awards

     4.   higher risk of musculoskeletal injury associated with high intensity training

     5.   not all highly trained competitors are physically fit

               a.   some excellent golfers and baseball players are overweight and lack good cardiorespiratory systems

    D.   Exercising for health
        1.   more moderate intensity
        2.   shorter bouts of activity
        3.   physiological benefits with less risk of injury

IV.   Health-related components of physical fitness
    A.   Cardiorespiratory endurance
        1.   the ability to perform large muscle movements over a sustained period of time
                a.   the ability of the circulatory (heart, blood, blood vessels) and respiratory (lungs, diaphragm, and so on) systems to deliver fuel, especially oxygen to the muscles during continuous exercise
        2.   cardiorespiratory endurance can be achieved through sustained large muscle movements such as brisk walking, jogging, swimming
                a.   health benefits include stronger heart, improved circulation to the heart, increased oxygen transportation by the blood, a lower risk of coronary heart attack, a decreased level of blood fat (cholesterol), increased level of high-density blood pressure, and a better chance of living a longer, healthier life

    B.   Body composition
        1.   refers to the relative amounts of lean body mass and fat in your body
                a.   lean body mass includes bones, muscles, and connective tissue
                b.   fat includes subcutaneous fat (fat deposits stored within the muscles)
        2.   the percentage of fat you have can be measured in several ways, including the skinfold technique and underwater weighing (hydrostatic weighing)
                a.   a certain amount of fat is essential for health, but too high or too low a percentage of fat is unhealthy
                b.   body composition can be improved by decreasing the amount of fat or increasing the amount of lean body mass or both
                        (1)   increasing muscle mass has the added advantage of increasing your resting metabolic rate
                c.   benefits of maintaining a healthy percentage of body fat include reducing your CHD risk, building an attractive physique, increasing your self-concept and improving your body's capacity to work.

    C.   Flexibility
        1.   is the ability to move a joint through its full range of motion
                a.   when muscle and connective tissue tighten and shorten, the range of motion in the joint is restrictive
                b.   too loose a joint can result in slippage, injury, and possible dislocation
        2.   you can work on flexibility by stretching during the warm-up or cool-down or by performing a specific flexibility program

    D.   Muscular Endurance
        1.   is the ability of a muscle or group of muscles to
                a.   apply submaximal (less than all-out) force repeatedly
                b.   sustain a muscular contraction for a period of time

    2.   you can improve muscular endurance by performing a relatively high number of repetitions of a movement against light to moderate resistance or by increasing the amount of time you hold a position

E.   Muscular Strength

    1.   is the ability of a muscle or group of muscles to exert force against a resistance

        a.   maximal strength is the amount of weight a person can move at one time

        b.   muscular strength is improved by lifting relatively heavy weights for a low number of repetitions

    2.   weight training is one of the best ways to increase strength

V.   How much physical activity is enough?

A.   In 1978 and 1990 ACSM published a set of guidelines on the recommended quantity and quality of exercise for healthy adults. The recommendations were based on research concerning how much exercise was needed for performance criteria.

    1.   the recommendations encouraged people to perform 20 to 60 minutes of moderate to high-intensity endurance exercise three to five times a week

    2.   people were also urged to perform a minimum of one set of eight to twelve repetitions of eight to ten exercises involving the major muscle groups twice a week

B.   More recently, research has looked at the amount of physical activity needed to acquire health benefits, as opposed to performance measures.

        a.   performing a lower intensity activity than previously recommended yields substantial benefits, especially among low fit or sedentary populations

        b.   health benefits raise quickly as inactive or low-active persons increase their activity to moderate level

        c.   moderate-level activities like a brisk 30-minute walk or three 10-minute sessions of serious activity will work

C.   In 1995 the CDC and ACSM published a set of physical activity guidelines.

    1.   meant to complement existing guidelines, not replace them

    2.   recommendations that every U.S. adult accumulate 30 minutes or more of moderately intense physical activity on most days of the week

        a.   moderately intense is equivalent of brisk walking (3 to 4 miles per hour for most adults)

        b.   physical activity can be categorized by the number of calories burned per unit of time

VI.   The benefits of physical activity and exercise are many.

A.   Thirty minutes of daily physical activity is the foundation of fitness and the minimum requirement for wellness

    1.   higher levels of fitness are achieved through vigorous cardiorespiratory activity and moderately challenging strength and muscular endurance exercises

    2.   high-intensity activities and competitive sports offer little additional advantage in terms of health benefits

B.   Social, emotional, spiritual and mental benefits

    1.   exercise is something most people enjoy doing with others

    2.   exercise lifts your spirit, particularly aerobic exercises

        a.   may help ease depression and reduce stress

          b.   aerobic exercise is believed to increase the number of endorphins circulating in your bloodstream

            (1)   endorphins are natural painkillers thought to be responsible for the euphoric feeling many people have after exercising

            (2)   this feeling is referred to as the "runner's high"

                (a)   not limited to running; any aerobic activity can produce it

                (b)   may take you six to eight weeks of doing regular exercise before you experience this "high"

    3.   spiritual insights may be gained through challenging physical activity

          a.   a healthy body frees you to concentrate on mental and spiritual events

    4.   lowering stress through physical activity may help clear your mind

  C.   Physical benefits

    1.   important influence on the five modifiable factors for coronary heart failure

          a.   a sedentary lifestyle is eliminated

          b.   high blood cholesterol and hypertension are lowered

          c.   cardiorespiratory system is improved

          d.   body fat decreases and obesity can in time be eliminated

          e.   exercise can help people quit smoking by acting as a substitute activity

VII.   Exercise and asthma

  A.   Asthma is a disease in which the muscles surrounding the airways constrict, causing shortness of breath, wheezing, and coughing.

    1.   allergies, infections, emotions and exercise can trigger an attack

    2.   exercise-induced asthma (EIA)

          a.   exercise improvements in the cardiorespiratory system raise the exertion level at which symptoms begin to occur

          b.   people with controlled asthma can and should exercise (in consultation with a physician)

            (1)   if you have EIA, try to recognize the symptoms early and lower your intensity or take a break

            (2)   if you use bronchodilator medication, keep it with you

            (3)   long gradual warm-ups and cool downs may ease the symptoms

            (4)   drink plenty of fluid and be careful on days in which the environmental conditions are more likely to trigger an attack

VIII. Exercise and diabetes

  A.   Diabetes is a metabolic disease in which the pancreas fails to produce sufficient insulin (Type I) or the body is unable to use the insulin it does produce (Type II).

    1.   insulin's role is to regulate the amount of sugar (glucose) in the blood

    2.   regular moderate exercise helps persons with diabetes maintain normal blood glucose levels and in some cases may reduce the need for insulin

  B.   Exercise guidelines include

    1.   avoiding exercise on an empty stomach

    2.   know when and where to take insulin shots

    3.   wearing good socks and keeping feet dry

    4.   trying to exercise at the same time of day

    5.   wearing a medical alert tag and telling friends

IX.   The metabolic systems: Turning food into energy

A.   Metabolic systems are often referred to as the body's energy system.
     1.   convert the food you eat into chemical energy
         a.   muscle cells then convert this chemical energy into mechanical energy to produce movement
         b.   different energy systems metabolize different nutrients
     2.   being able to match exercises and foods with energy systems will help you know how to lose fat and how to gain muscle
         a.   food is digested and chemically processed to produce adenosine triphosphate (ATP), a high-energy phosphate molecule that, when split, releases energy for your body's cells
         b.   muscle cells use ATP to fuel the contraction process
         c.   movement is possible as long as ATP is available
             (1)   rigor mortis occurs when ATP is not available

B.   Anaerobic metabolism
     1.   means "without oxygen"
         a.   during short, intense bursts of activity, the body cannot meet the muscles' demand for oxygen
         b.   the body is equipped with two energy-producing systems that do not depend on oxygen
             (1)   phosphagen system
             (2)   lactic acid system
         c.   these anaerobic systems are rapid sources of ATP for short periods of time
     2.   phosphagen system
         a.   most rapid anaerobic system
             (1)   this form of stored energy is used to get you going at the beginning of exercise, especially if you start quickly
             (2)   small amounts of high-energy phosphagens are stored directly in the muscle cells
                 (a)   as ATP is broken down, the high-energy phosphagen builds it back up
             (3)   the muscle can store only enough high-energy phosphagen to produce ATP for one to six seconds of activity
             (4)   this system is not very important for lifetime fitness
             (5)   as the phosphagen system is depleted, the lactic acid system takes over as the main energy producer
     3.   lactic acid system
         a.   the lactic acid system produces ATP by breaking down carbohydrates (glucose) without oxygen
             (1)   along with energy, lactic acid and heat are produced
                 (a)   the heat dissipates through sweat
                 (b)   with intense anaerobic activity, lactic acid build up makes the muscle feel heavy and "burn"
                 (c)   when exercise stops or is reduced to a lower intensity, the concentration of lactic acid decreases

                (2)   after exercise, breathing continues to be deep and rapid until enough oxygen has been delivered to clear up the lactic acid and return the cardiorespiratory system to homeostasis

        b.   activities that depend on anaerobic metabolism for energy are usually short, intense and powerful

              (1)   predominantly anaerobic activities last for less than a minute

        c.   anaerobic glycolysis also plays a major role in intense activities that last for one to three minutes

              (1)   many activities are partly anaerobic and partly aerobic

     d.   exercise benefits associated with anaerobic training include muscular strength and endurance and cardiorespiratory fitness

C.   Aerobic metabolism

     1.   aerobic means "with oxygen"

     2.   breaks down carbohydrates (aerobic glycolysis) and fat (fatty acid oxidation) in the presence of oxygen to produce ATP, carbon dioxide, water and heat

        a.   carbon dioxide is transported by the blood to the lungs, where it is exhaled from the body

        b.   heat and water are released primarily through sweat

     3.   carbohydrates are the primary source of fuel for the aerobic system

        a.   when the body will have to meet an elevated energy demand for a long time, it will conserve carbohydrates and use fat

              (1)   burning fat is called fatty acid oxidation, also called beta oxidation

     4.   fatty acid oxidation must be coaxed into operation

        a.   to benefit from this process, exercise for at least 20 minutes

        b.   to burn fat, exercise for a longer period of time at a moderate intensity than for a short time at a high intensity

              (1)   high-intensity activity primarily burns carbohydrates, whereas low to moderate-intensity burns both fat and carbohydrates

              (2)   low-intensity activities tend to burn a high percentage of fat, but also fewer calories per minute than moderate-intensity activities

     5.   fat and carbohydrates are both being burned at rest and during exercise, but the percentage of each and the overall consumption of each vary with the intensity of activity

     6.   aerobic exercises are continuous, rhythmic activities using large-muscle groups

        a.   health benefits associated with aerobic activities include cardiorespiratory endurance, weight management, and muscle endurance

X.   Getting off to a good start

    A.   Medical clearance

       1.   a thorough medical examination with a stress test performed by a physician is recommended for males over 40, females over 50, or anyone with a chronic disease or risk factor for chronic disease

    B.   Dressing for physical activity

       1.   wear nonrestrictive clothing that allows heat and moisture to escape

       2.   wear supportive undergarments

       3.   wear layers of clothing so that you can peel off layers as you get hot and add layers as you get cold

4. wear comfortable and supportive shoes
5. the type of clothing and corresponding equipment will vary a great deal, depending on the activities you select
6. seek out an expert for activity-specific needs

C. Goal setting
1. decide what it is you want to do—general goal
2. assess where you are right now
3. make your general goal more specific, using information from your assessment
4. decide how you are going to accomplish your goal
5. add a time frame
6. write a very specific goal incorporating all the information from the first five steps
7. decide how you will evaluate and monitor your progress

IX. Planning an exercise session
A. Components of a physical activity session
1. warm-up
   a. first part of a warm-up consists of a series of movements and stretches to warm and prepare the body for activity
   b. start off slowly and gradually build up to a brisk pace
      (1) first, easy, active movements
      (2) work up to a moderate pace, one vigorous enough to raise body temperature and increase circulation but not so fast that momentum carries the limbs beyond comfortable range of motion
      (3) as muscles warm up, they become more elastic; warm muscles are also capable of more forceful and rapid movements than cold muscles and are less vulnerable to injury
   c. warm-up activity signals the release of synovial fluid
      (1) this fluid, secreted into the joints, acts as a lubricant
   d. the second part of the warm-up is stretching exercises
2. the workout
   a. the workout is the main activity for which the warm-up has prepared you
   b. an exercise workout might include one or more of the following components
      (1) flexibility
      (2) muscle strengthening
      (3) muscle endurance
      (4) cardiorespiratory endurance
   c. a workout can be defined by three variables: frequency (F), intensity (I), and time (T), known as the FIT Principle
      (5) a minimum amount and intensity of exercise must be performed before fitness improvements begin; this minimum level of exercise is called the threshold of training
      (6) the optimal intensity range for exercise is called the fitness target zone
         (a) the lower limit of the zone is the threshold of training; the upper limit is the maximum amount of exercise that is beneficial

         (b)   the best known target zone is the one for cardiorespiratory endurance

    d.   performing more than one activity is called cross training

    e.   cross training offers people the advantage of variety and of working different muscles or the same muscles in different ways

3.   cool-down

    a.   the cool down is the activity that follows the workout; its purpose is to bring the body gradually back down to a resting state

    b.   the actual movements and techniques required for the cool-down are just like the warm-up, only you reverse the process

    c.   helps return the blood to the heart for re-oxygenation (venous pump)

4.   developmental stretch is the last segment of an activity session.

    a.   the purpose is to relieve muscle tension and develop flexibility

        (7)   same stretches and stretch techniques used during the warm-up are used for the closing stretch with one exception, that the stretches should be held longer

XII.   Exercise and pregnancy

    A.   Exercise is a positive health habit that in most cases can be continued through pregnancy.

        5.   it is best to start an exercise program before pregnancy, but it is certainly possible to begin with light exercising during pregnancy

        6.   pregnant women or women considering pregnancy should discuss an exercise plan with their physician

    B.   The American College of Obstetricians and Gynecologists (ACOG) has published exercise guidelines for healthy pregnant women.

XIII.   Principles of physical activity

    A.   Principle of individuality

        7.   holds that no two people react exactly the same way to exercise

        8.   when comparing self against fitness test norms, averages, or percentiles, keep in mind your individuality

        9.   put more emphasis on improving your own scores than comparing scores

    B.   Principle of overload

        10.   holds that improvement occurs when something is done to a greater extent than normal

        11.   involves an increase in frequency, intensity, or time

          a.   as your body adapts, a training effect occurs

          b.   when a desired level of fitness is reached, overloading can be stopped

            (8)   to maintain your fitness level, continue to perform your new normal amount

        12.   overuse is a result of violating the principle of overload

    C.   Principle of progression

        13.   holds that overloads should be performed gradually over time

          a.   too slow a progression does not result in optimum training

          b.   too fast a progression may result in excessive soreness and injury

        14.   the phrase "progressive overload" is often used to describe the application of this principle

    D.   Principle of specificity

15   holds that placing a specific demand on the body results in a specific adaptation

16   select exercises that will result in the desired outcome

  E.   Principle of reversibility

      17.   basic tenet is "use it or lose it"

      18.   sometimes referred to as detraining or the use-disuse principle

         a.   exercise/physical activity must be ongoing to maintain a level of fitness

XIV. Maintaining an exercise program

  A.   Adherence to exercise programs is often poor.

  B.   Thirty to seventy percent of those who start drop out within six months.

  C.   To increase chances of adherence, choose activities that

      19.   are enjoyable

      20.   can be done near home, work, or campus

      21.   are financially comfortable

      22.   are supported by family and friends

      23.   are natural extensions of your daily routine

  D.   Assessment

      24.   tracking progress can be very motivational

      25.   physical fitness can be assessed using expensive equipment in established exercise laboratories or through fairly simple field tests

XV. Injury prevention and care

  A.   When injury occurs and the cause of the injury can be identified , the activity, the equipment being used, or the environment in which the activity is performed can often be modified to eliminate or minimize the risk of injury.

      26.   work to correct foot-plant technique errors that may be causing the problem

      27.   purchase better shock-absorbing shoes

      28.   run on more even surfaces

      29.   change to a nonimpact activity like cycling

  B.   Strong and flexible muscles can prevent many injuries.

  C.   See Appendix C in the text for the prevention and care of common injuries.

BEHAVIOR BOOSTS—STUDENT ACTIVITIES

- Surround yourself with supportive people: workout buddies, family members, exercise class members.
- Try to establish a regular exercise time that won't be easily interrupted.
- Get your workout clothes and equipment ready ahead of time.
- Do something you enjoy.
- Plan vacations that include fun physical activities.
- Treat yourself to a reward for sticking with your program.
- Acknowledge the importance of physical activity/exercise and give it priority.
- Change activities or use a variety of activities (cross train) if you are getting bored.
- Change locations: take your bike to a new trail or country road, walk a new path or reverse your normal route, swim in a lake during the summer instead of doing laps in a pool.
- Train for competition: check your recreation clubs or intramural groups.

·   Teach physical activity: community, youth, and senior citizen groups, and Special Olympics programs need volunteers.
·   Put home exercise equipment in front of the TV or in a place where you tend to sit and socialize.

ADDITIONAL STUDENT ACTIVITIES

Activity 1: Calculating Minutes of Moderate Intensity Exercise

Use Activity 2.1 on page 31 of the text to determine how long you will need to perform a type of activity to burn the calories you wish to burn.

Activity 2: Par-Q & You

Fill out the Par-Q form on page 37 of the text and follow up with a visit to a doctor if indicated.

Activity 3: Are Your Activities Aerobic or Anaerobic?

List the physical activities you are presently engaged in or are considering starting in the near future. Then identify whether these activities are primarily aerobic, anaerobic, or a combination of both. List the criteria you used for your choices. For example, tennis is both aerobic and anaerobic because a match takes 1–3 hours of continuous play (aerobic), but within that time there are short intense actions followed by long breaks (anaerobic). Now decide if the activities you engage in help you meet your fitness goals.

Activity 4: Applying the Components and Principles of Physical Activity

Think of one exercise or sport activity and one non-exercise-related activity. Plan a session for each using the components of physical activity (warm-up, workout, cool-down). Outline what you would do for each component.

For each example above, identify how each of the principles of physical activity was incorporated or considered.

LABS

None—see each of the chapters on health-related components of physical fitness.

ADDITIONAL INFORMATION

Quick tips for building moderately-intense physical activity into your day.

·   Park your car at a distance from your destination and walk at a brisk pace.
·   Walk or play with a pet.
·   Play sports or an active game like hide and seek with a friend or child.

- Take the stairs at the library, mall, airport, or at home.
- Go dancing or dance around the house.
- Get off the bus or subway one stop early and walk.
- Clean your room or house.
- Do yard work (or house work) for yourself, a church, an elderly or sick friend.
- Garden.
- Build something.
- Deliver bills, gifts, food, or information in person instead of sending them by fax or through the mail.
- Place exercise equipment in front of the television set and use it while watching a favorite show.
- Join an informal or formal exercise group.
- Wear clothing to picnics and other social gatherings that allow you to spontaneously join in activities like Frisbee, volleyball, or horseshoes.
- Teach someone how to play a game or sport.
- Walk to someone's room or house instead of phoning.

RESOURCES

Suggested Reading

American College of Sports Medicine. *Guidelines for exercise testing and prescription*, 4th ed. Philadelphia: Lea & Febiger, 1991.

American College of Sports Medicine. The recommended quantity and quality of exercise for developing and maintaining cardiorespiratory and muscular fitness in healthy adults. *Medicine and Science in Sports* 22(2):265-274, 1990.

Brunick, T. Choosing the right shoe. *The Physician and Sportsmedicine* 18(7):104, 1990.

Fletcher, G.F., et al. American Heart Association: Statement on exercise. *Circulation* 862726, 1992.

Healthy people 2000 objectives and the national education goals. *Public Health Reports* 107(1):10-15, 1992.

International Society of Sport Psychology. *Physical activity and psychological benefits*: Position statement 20:179, 1992.

Paffenbarger, R.S., Jr., R.T. Hyde, A.L. Wing, and C.C. Hsieh. Physical activity, all-cause mortality, and longevity of college alumni. *New England Journal of Medicine* 314:605-613, 1986.

Pate, R.R., et al. Physical activity and public health: A recommendation from the Centers for Disease Control and Prevention and the American College of Sports Medicine. *Journal of the American Medical Association* 273(5):402-407, 1995.

Shepard, R.J. *Aerobic fitness & health*. Champaign, IL: Human Kinetics, 1994.

U.S. Department of Health and Human Services. *Physical activity and health: A report of the Surgeon General*. Centers for Disease Control and Prevention, National Centers for Chronic Disease Prevention and Health Promotion. Atlanta: The President's Council on Physical Fitness and Sports, 1996.

U.S. Department of Health and Human Services. *Healthy people 2000*: National health promotion and disease prevention objectives. DHHS Publication No (PHS) 91-50213. Washington, D.C.: U.S. Government Printing Office, 1990.

University of California at Berkeley. *The New Wellness Encyclopedia*, Boston: Houghton Mifflin, 1995.

Williams, M. *Lifetime Fitness and Wellness*, W.C. Brown, Dubuque, IA, 1996.

Wilmore, J.H. and D.L. Costill. *Training for sport and activity: The physiological basis of the conditioning process*, 3rd ed. Champaign, IL: Human Kinetics, 1993.

Organizations

Aerobic and Fitness Association of America
(AFAA)
15250 Ventura Blvd., Suite 892
Sherman Oaks, CA 91403
Tel (800) 225-2322
Fax (818) 990-5468
Web site: http://www.aerobics.com

American Alliance of Health, Physical Education,
Recreation and Dance (AAHPERD)
1900 Association Drive
Reston, VA 20191-1599
Tel (800) 213-7193
E-mail: info@aahperd.org
Web site: http://www.aahperd.org

American Academy of Allergy, Asthma, &
Immunology
611 East Wells Street
Milwaukee, WI 53202
Tel (414) 272-6071
Web site: http://www.AAAAI.org

American College of Sports Medicine (ACSM)
P.O. Box 1440
Indianapolis, IN 46206-1440
Tel (317) 637-9200
Fax (317) 634-7817
Web site: http://www.acsm.org

American College of Surgeons
633 North Saint Clair Street
Chicago, IL 60611-3211
Tel (312) 202-5000
Fax (312) 202-5001
Web site: http://www.facs.org

American Council on Exercise (ACE)
6190 Cornerstone Court, East, Suite 202
San Diego, CA 92121-4729
5820 Oberlin Drive, Suite 102
San Diego, CA 92121-3787
Tel (619) 535-8227
Fax (619) 535-1778
Web site: http://www.ACEfitness.org

American Diabetes Association
1660 Duke Street
Alexandria, VA 22314
Tel: see web site for local phone numbers
Web site: http://www.diabetes.org

The American Dietetic Association
216 West Jackson Boulevard
Chicago, IL 60606-6995
Tel (312) 899-0040
Fax (312) 899-1979
Web site: http://www.eatright.org

American Heart Association
National Center
7272 Greenville Avenue
Dallas, TX 75231
Tel (800) AHA-USA1 (Customer Heart & Stroke Information)
Tel (888) MY-HEART (Women's Health Information)
Web site: http://www.aha.org

American Medical Athletic Association (AMAA)
4405 East West Highway, Suite 405
Bethesda, MD 20804
Tel: (800) 776-2732
Web site: http://www.arfa.org/amaa

Association for Fitness in Business
865 Hope Street
Stamford, CT 06907
(203) 359-2188

Cooper Institute for Aerobic Research (CIAR)
12330 Preston Road
Dallas, TX 75230
Tel (800) 635-7050
Fax (972) 341-3224
Web site: http://www.cooperinst.org

Food and Nutrition Information Center
Web site: http://www.nalusda.gov/fnic

IDEA
6190 Cornerstone Court East, Suite 204
San Diego, CA 92121-3773
Tel (800) 999-4332 ext. 7
Tel (619) 535-8979 ext. 7
Fax (619) 535-8234
Home page: http://www.ideafit.com

Jewish Community Centers of America
Web site: www.jcca.org

President's Council on Physical Fitness and Sports (PCPFS)
450 Fifth Street, NW, Suite 7103

Washington, DC 20001
(202) 272-2451
Web site: http://www.hhs.gov/progorg/ophs/pcpfs

Rockport Walking Institute
220 Donald Lynch Blvd.
Marlboro, MA 01752
Tel (800) rockport (762-5767)
Web site: http://www.rockport.com

U.S. Department of Agriculture
14th & Independence Avenue SW
Washington, DC 20250
Tel (202) 720-2791
Web site: http://www.usda.gov

YMCA of the USA
101 North Wacker Drive
Chicago, IL 60606
Tel: (312) 977-0031
Fax: (312) 977-9063
Web site: www.ymca.net

YWCA of the USA
Empire State Building
Suite 301
New York, NY 10118
Tel: (212) 275-0800
Fax: (212) 465-2281
Web site: www.ywca. org

Video

How fit are you? YMCA Program Store, Box 5077, Champaign, IL 61820.

Additional Local and Community Resources

American Heart Association
Blue Cross/Blue Shield
County Recreation Departments
Governor's Council on Health and Fitness
State and County Health Departments

Cardiorespiratory Endurance

Chapter 3

CHAPTER SUMMARY

Cardiorespiratory endurance may be the most important health-related component of fitness due to its large impact on coronary heart disease risk factors and other chronic diseases. It provides us with stamina and extra energy for recreational activities. Aerobic training provides stress release and may result in the euphoric "runner's high." Physical activity at a moderate intensity for 30 minutes a day provides substantial disease protection and improves health, while vigorous activity promotes a higher level of fitness and physical performance.

To improve aerobic fitness you must exercise above your aerobic threshold and within your aerobic target zone. The target zone is described by the FIT variables: frequency, intensity, time. Optimum cardiorespiratory fitness occurs when you exercise three to five times a week, at 60 to 80 percent of heart rate reserve, for 20 to 60 minutes. Beginners should work at the lower end of the target zone, while more fit individuals can work out at intensities near the high end.

LEARNING OBJECTIVES

The student will be able to:

- describe the health benefits associated with cardiorespiratory activity
- explain the physiological impact of physical activity on the cardiorespiratory system.
- describe the target zone for aerobic exercise in terms of frequency, intensity , and time.
- calculate and monitor a target heart rate zone.
- assess cardiorespiratory endurance and set appropriate goals for improvement or maintenance.
- establish an activity plan—either for a formal exercise program or for informal daily physical activities.
- dress and exercise safely in the heat, cold, and high altitude.

PERSONAL PROFILE

Arnold Schwarzenegger

Arnold Schwarzenegger might be one of the hottest movie stars around, but there is more to Arnold than muscles and tough-guy movies. The world's most famous muscleman has been on a mission to promote fitness across America. The Austrian-born actor came to the United States at the age of twenty-one determined to accomplish his goal of becoming the best body builder in the world. He did this and more and turned his attention to a different goal: bringing daily physical education classes back into the schools. In 1989 he was appointed chairman of the President's Council on Physical Education and Sport, where he promoted fitness and regular exercise across America.

Besides meeting with every governor in the nation, Arnold made numerous stops at schools, universities, and press conferences, where he met with legislators, students, and fitness professionals to convince them of the need for regular aerobic exercise. At one elementary school assembly, Arnold told the children, "Don't just sit there in front of the TV and stuff yourself with junk food. Ride your bicycle, go hiking, or at least do pushups and sit-ups." His message is clear: Get up and exercise.

So what does Arnold do in his personal exercise program? For one thing, Arnold has to weight train for an hour each day just to maintain the muscle mass needed for body building, but he doesn't stop there. Each day Arnold does at least thirty minutes of aerobic exercise to help him stay fit. His favorite sports are tennis, hiking, and skiing. In addition, his exercise routine is accompanied by a diet low in fat, and high in fruits and vegetables. A wellness lifestyle helps him succeed in all that he does because for Arnold, "the joy of life is not just to exist, but to take on new challenges." It looks as if Arnold understands what wellness is all about.

Krucoff, Carol. Pumping Arnold. American Health, 10(1)44-49, 1992.

CONTENT OUTLINE

I. What is cardiorespiratory endurance?
   A. The ability of the cardiovascular and respiratory systems to provide fuel, especially oxygen, to the muscles and the ability of the muscles to use this fuel for sustained physical work.
      1. aerobic exercise is the preferred type of exercise for increasing cardiorespiratory endurance
         a. because it specifically trains the cardiovascular, respiratory, and muscular systems to better consume , transport, and use oxygen
      2. anaerobic exercise also contributes to cardiorespiratory endurance by improving the delivery of oxygen in the blood, increasing blood flow, and strengthening the heart
         a. anaerobic exercise does not improve muscle cells' ability to use the oxygen to produce more energy
         b. to benefit from anaerobic training you must train at very high all-out intensity efforts for short amounts of time alternated with short rest periods
      3. people prefer to train their cardiorespiratory system using aerobic exercise
         a. the moderate intensity and continuous nature of aerobic conditioning tends to be more comfortable and therefore more enjoyable
            (1) provides fitness base that supports daily and recreational activities
            (2) anaerobic training is more performance-oriented and is therefore more important for those training for competitive sports
         b. to attain a moderate to high level of cardiorespiratory endurance, you must exercise vigorously enough to produce a training effect

II.   Heart: The system's pump
    A.   Four-chambered organ composed of cardiac muscle that controls the volume and speed at which oxygen and other nutrients are delivered to the working muscles.
        1.   heart rate (HR): rate of contraction
        2.   stroke volume (SV): the amount of blood ejected from the heart per beat
        3.   cardiac output (CO): amount of blood pumped out of the heart per minute   (HR x SV)
        4.   during exertion HR and SV increase to increase delivery of oxygen
            a.   most of the increase is in HR
    B.   Benefits of Exercise
        1.   cardiac (heart) muscle becomes stronger with exercise
            a.   left ventricle (chamber that ejects blood into the body) adapts differently depending on the kind of physical training performed
                (1)   anaerobic training: the walls thicken
                (2)   aerobic training: the volume of the chamber increases
            b.   the heart can pump more blood with each beat or the same amount of blood with fewer beats
        2.   stroke volume increases
            a.   average resting stroke volume is 70 to 90 milliliters per beat
            b.   during exercise the stroke volume can increase to 100 to 120 milliliters per beat
        3.   resting heart rate (RHR) decreases
            a.   increased strength and volume allows heart to pump more blood with fewer beats
            b.   the average resting heart rate is 70–80 bpm
            c.   with regular aerobic exercise the bpm can drop 10 to 20 bpm or more
            d.   aerobically fit individuals may have resting heart rates of 50–60 bpm
            e.   heredity also plays a role in establishing the resting heart rate
            f.   the resting heart rate is influenced not only by the strength of the heart
III.   Arteries: Pipelines of the system.
    A.   large arteries branch off into smaller and smaller arteries
        1.   the smallest arteries called capillaries deliver oxygen to the cells
        2.   the heart cells receive oxygen-rich blood through the two coronary arteries
    B.   Benefits of exercise
        1.   exercise increases the number of capillaries
            a.   allows better oxygen and carbon dioxide exchange
            b.   if blood flow is blocked, blood can be diverted to other healthy branches
                (1)   in the heart this means that if one pathway is blocked, oxygen-rich blood can be rerouted and delivered to the heart muscle; helps prevent ischemia and heart attacks
                (2)   in the brain, the greater network of arterial capillaries helps prevent a stroke
        2.   regular physical activity and a good diet can help prevent arterial diseases, lower blood pressure and decrease the levels of fat in the blood

        a.   blood pressure stays in a healthy range during exertion because healthy arteries stretch and can handle the extra blood flow

    3.   exercise increases the number of HDL (good cholesterol) which helps carry fat out of the bloodstream

IV.   Blood: The system's carrier

    A.   Blood performs a number of critical functions, including the transportation of oxygen and carbon dioxide.

        1.   microscopically, blood is composed of solids (red and white blood cells and platelets) and plasma (a liquid containing dissolved substances)

              a.   hemoglobin in the red blood cells combines with oxygen and carbon dioxide and transports them through the blood vessels

    B.   Benefits of exercise

        1.   blood volume increases in response to regular aerobic exercise

              a.   most of the increase is due to increase in blood plasma

              b.   this lowers the viscosity of the blood, which allows the blood to flow with less resistance, which lowers blood pressure

        2.   red blood cells and hemoglobin increase

              a.   greater oxygen and carbon dioxide capacity

              b.   muscle cells become more effective at extracting oxygen and other nutrients from the blood in the capillaries

V.   Lungs: The blood's oxygen depot

    A.   When you breathe in, you draw oxygen through the trachea and down the bronchial tubes into the lungs.

        1.   the bronchi branch repeatedly and eventually become small alveolar ducts

              a.   at the end of the ducts are numerous alveoli and alveolar sacs

              b.   between these alveoli and the tiny arteries and veins, oxygen and carbon dioxide are exchanged

    B.   Benefits of Exercise

        1.   respiratory muscles strengthen; therefore, pulmonary ventilation increases

              a.   average untrained person can ventilate about 120 liters of air per minute

              b.   pulmonary ventilation increases to about 150 liters of air following fitness training, and highly trained athletes can ventilate more than 180 liters per minute

VI.   Metabolic Process: The power plant.

    A.   Anaerobic processes take place in the cytoplasm of the muscle cell.

    B.   Aerobic processes take place inside the mitochondrion, a floating structure in the cytoplasm.

        1.   mitochondrion is often referred to as the "powerhouse" of the cells

              a.   inside this little "factory" simple sugars (carbohydrates after digestion) are converted into cellular energy (ATP)

    C.   Benefits of exercise

        1.   aerobic exercise increases the number of mitochondria and enzymes responsible for fat utilization

              a.   makes more energy available for physical activity

              b.   more fat can be mobilized

        2.   anaerobic conditioning results in greater storage of glycogen and high-energy phosphagens (ATP and CP) inside the muscle cells

        a.   the more energy a cell can store and/or produce, the longer an activity can be sustained

VII. Other benefits of aerobic exercise

    A.   It has a positive influence on social, emotional, and mental well-being.

    B.   It helps alleviate some depression, anxiety, and insomnia.

    C.   It decreases the secretion of hormones triggered by stress and provides an emotional outlet for pent-up anger.

VIII. How to improve cardiorespiratory endurance: The FIT principle

    A.   Frequency (FIT)

        1.   optimal aerobic training occurs when you exercise three to five times a week

            a.   the majority of improvements in aerobic capacity occur with three days of exercise a week

            b.   some additional improvements occur with four or five days of training

                (1)   after five days of training, improvements plateau

                (2)   exercising six or seven days results in little or no improvement, except in weight loss

        2.   exercise addicts are people who feel compelled to workout every single day

            a.   can suffer from overuse injuries, such as shinsplints, tendinitis

            b.   addiction to exercise, like any addiction, can lead to an unhealthy lifestyle

    B.   Intensity (FIT)

        1.   The higher the intensity of exercise, the more oxygen muscles need.

            a.   breathing becomes faster and deeper to bring in more oxygen, and the heart beats faster to speed up oxygen delivery to the muscles

            b.   as exercise intensity increases, the rate and volume of oxygen being consumed increases until the body is consuming oxygen as rapidly as it can

                (1)   this maximum volume of oxygen consumption (measured in liters per minute or milliliters per minute per kilogram body weight) is called VO_2max

                (2)   exercise above VO_2max is anaerobic and can only be performed for a short time before exhaustion occurs

                (3)   age, heredity, and physical training influence VO_2max

        2.   ACSM recommends that the normal healthy adult exercise aerobically at an intensity between 50 and 85 percent of VO_2max.

            a.   50 percent of VO_2max is called the threshold of training

            b.   most health-related exercise is performed at 60–80% of VO_2max

            c.   oxygen consumption is measured with scientific equipment which is not practical for everyday use

        3.   Heart rate has an almost linear relationship to oxygen consumption and can therefore be used to estimate oxygen consumption and monitor exercise intensity.

            a.   HR is determined by counting the pulse

            b.   maximum heart rate (MHR) is the fastest the heart can beat

            c.   ACSM recommends exercises between 60 and 90 percent of MHR

            d.   60–90% of MHR is equivalent to 50–85% of VO_2max

            e.   most health-related exercise is performed at 70–85% MHR

4. The training heart rate range (THR) is the range of heart rates that coincides with aerobic conditioning.
    a. often referred to as the target heart rate zone
    b. exercise keeping HR within the THR improves aerobic fitness
    c. range for health-related fitness is usually set in the middle of the ACSM ranges for cardiorespiratory conditioning:
        (1) 50–85% VO_2max ==> 60–80% VO_2max
        (2) 60–90 % MHR ==> 70–85% MHR
5. calculating the THR
    a. Maximum Heart Rate Formula
        (1) MHR = 220 - age
        (2) MHR x .60 = threshold of training
        (3) MHR x .80 = upper limit of range
    b. Karvonen formula
        (1) MHR = 220 - age
        (2) MHR - RHR X .60 + RHR = threshold of training
        (3) MHR - RHR x .80 + RHR = upper limit of range
6. exercise heart rate (EHR)
    a. the speed at which your heart is beating during exercise
        (1) EHR should fall within the THR
            (a) if EHR is higher than THR, exercise intensity is too high
            (b) if EHR is below the THR, exercise is not intense enough
    b. to find your EHR
        (1) count the pulse for 10 seconds while exercising or for 10 seconds within 15 seconds of the time you stop
7. taking your pulse
    a. press with a light to medium pressure on a main artery with two fingers (not your thumb)
    b. two most common arteries for taking pulse
        (1) carotid artery located just to the side of your larynx
            (a) in some people may cause dizziness or slowing of the pulse
        (2) radial artery located on the inside of your wrist
    c. count for 10 seconds
8. ratings of perceived exertion (RPE)
    a. Gunnar Borg discovered a relationship between perception of exercise intensity and heart rate
        (1) developed the ratings of perceived exertion (RPE) scale
        (2) RPE works when heart rate is not reliable
            (a) if you are on medication that affects heart rate, or are not good at taking your pulse
9. talk test
    a. you should be able to talk comfortable while working out
        (1) if you cannot. your workout is too intense
        (2) if you can sing comfortably. your intensity is probably too low
10. when to monitor intensity
    a. monitor level of exertion periodically during the workout

        (1)   5 to 10 minutes into an aerobic workout to make certain you have reached your training intensity

        (2)   at the peak, to make certain you are not too high

        (3)   at the end of the aerobic workout, to check to see if you maintained the training intensity to the end

C.   Time (FIT)

    1.   ACSM describes the optimal duration of cardiorespiratory workout as 20 to 60 minutes.

       a.   is a guideline; adjustments should be made according to the activity and fitness level of the individual

       b.   Dr. Cooper recommends running be limited to 80 to 90 minutes a week, at three times a week for 30 minutes or four times a week for 20 minutes (prevention of overuse injuries)

       c.   performing any kind of aerobic activity for more than 60 minutes brings diminishing returns

IX.   Applying the principles of physical activity/exercise to cardiorespiratory endurance

    A.   Principles of progression and overload

       1.   increase intensity after achieving the appropriate frequency and duration

       2.   goal of 30 minutes moderately intense physical activity or 20 minutes of vigorous exercise

    B.   Principle of individuality

       1.   select activities that meet your needs and interests

       2.   fat loss will occur in different places and at different rates for different people

       3.   RHR will decline at different rates and amounts for different people

       4.   beginners will show more dramatic cardiorespiratory fitness improvements but everyone can improve

    C.   Principle of specificity

       1.   aerobic activities of sufficient intensity encourage fat mobilization and are less likely to cause musculoskeletal injury than anaerobic activities

    D.   Principle of reversibility

       1.   cardiorespiratory health benefits are maintained only as long as you stay active

X.   Designing your cardiorespiratory program

    A.   When setting up a program for improving your cardiorespiratory endurance, the following steps can be useful.

       1.   assess your present level of cardiorespiratory fitness

         a.   write a general goal

       2.   select one or more cardiorespiratory activities for your program

       3.   determine the frequency, intensity, and duration to perform your chosen activity or activities

         a.   write one or more specific goals

       4.   set a date to begin

         a.   sign up for an activity

XI.   Exercise and the environment

    A.   Take into account the environment in which you will be active.

       1.   air, noise, and water pollution

        a.   check with authorities for safe water, air condition, etc.

        b.   exercise in the morning when air is the cleanest

2.   hot and sunny weather

        a.   dress appropriately

        b.   stay well hydrated

        c.   use sunblock and wear a hat/sunglasses

3.   cold weather

        a.   dress in layers

        b.   wear sunglasses and sunblock

        c.   stay hydrated and eat to stay warm

        d.   make sure someone knows where you are going

4.   high altitude

        a.   start slowly

        b.   stay well hydrated

        c.   avoid alcohol and sleeping pills

        d.   if altitude sick, rest and see a physician

BEHAVIOR BOOSTS: STAGE-BASED STUDENT ACTIVITIES

Precontemplator
- Make a note of any time you feel winded or have to stop doing something to catch your breath.
- Stop and think if there is anything you'd like to do, but don't, because it causes you discomfort or because you lack the stamina.
- Determine how many risk factors you have for CHD and how many of those risks can be reduced or eliminated through regular physical activity. (Turn to Lab 9.1 to determine CHD risk.)

Contemplator
- Make a list of physical activities you would enjoy doing.
- Think about where and when you could do the activities you enjoy.
- If you are employed, find out if your job benefits include things that make exercising easier, such as workout facility, or flex time.
- Examine the fitness tests in the Labs in this chapter and think about which one you would be willing to try.
- Identify people in your social group who exercise and consider joining one or more of them.

Preparer
- Select and jot down one to three activities you would enjoy doing.
- Purchase or prepare any equipment or clothing you need to participate in at least one activity involving exercise. (Walking is very inexpensive; you just need comfortable shoes and loose clothing.)
- Set a date to begin exercising and post it somewhere highly visible.
- Find a friend who will join you in an activity involving exercise.
- Sign up for physical activity at your college (course , club sports or intramurals), YMCA/YWCA or recreation department.

Action Taker

Moderately Intense Cardiorespiratory Activity
- Walk at a brisk pace, with your thoughts, with a pet, with a friend, to a friend's house.
- Walk up twenty flights of stairs each day. (Or do fewer flights and combine with another activity.)
- Walk or cycle to campus, or work, or to do errands.
- Go dancing, or dance around the house.
- Get off the bus or subway one stop early and walk.
- Go hiking, rowing, swimming, or cycling at a moderate intensity.
- Mow the lawn with a push mower.
- Use exercise equipment (treadmill, stair-stepper) at a moderate intensity.

Vigorous Cardiorespiratory Activity
- Play one or more cardiorespiratory-demanding sports, including soccer (not as goalie), hockey, racket sports, lacrosse, swimming, water polo, or running.
- Participate in a vigorous aerobic activity, such as jogging, cycling, swimming, inline skating, cross-country skiing.
- Exercise vigorously using aerobic exercise equipment, such as a stair stepper, treadmill, stationary bike, slide board, or aerobic step.

Maintainer
- Vary your activities—cross train to prevent boredom.
- Invite others to join you.
- Make a plan for how you will maintain your activity level during holidays, business trips, or stressful times such as finals week.
- Sign up for a class with an instructor who shows concern when you miss a class.
- Practice injury prevention (Chapter 2) and seek medical advice when you are injured or think you may be developing a chronic injury like tendinitis or shinsplints.

ADDITIONAL STUDENT ACTIVITIES

Activity 1: Find Your Target Heart Rate Zone

Using the worksheet on text page 54, calculate your target heart rate zone.

LABS

Lab 3.1 What Can I Do? (pages 61–63)
Lab 3.2 One-Mile Rockport Walk Test (pages 64–65)
Lab 3.3 12-Minute Swim Test (page 66)
Lab 3.4 1.5-Mile Timed Run Test (page 67)
Lab 3.5 Developing Your Cardiorespiratory Endurance Program (pages 68–69)

RESOURCES

Suggested Reading

American College of Sports Medicine. The recommended quantity and quality of exercise for developing and maintaining cardiorespiratory and muscular fitness in healthy adults. *Medicine and Science in Sports* 22(2):265-274, 1990.

American Heart Association. *The healthy-heart walking book: The American Heart Association Walking Program.* New York: Macmillan, 1993.

Cooper, K.H. *The aerobics program for total well-being.* New York: M. Evans, 1982.

DeLorne, R. and F. Stransky. *Fitness and Fallacies.* Dubuque, Iowa: Kendall/Hunt, 1990.

Dishman, R.K., ed. *Advances in exercise adherence.* Champaign, IL: Human Kinetics, 1994.

Iknoian, T. *Fitness walking technique, motivation, and 60 workouts for walkers (fitness spectrum).* Champaign, IL: Human Kinetics, 1995.

Pate, R.R., et al. Physical activity and public health: A recommendation from the Centers for Disease Control and Prevention and the American College of Sports Medicine. *Journal of the American Medical Association* 273(5):402-407, 1995.

Powers, S., and E. Howley. *Exercise physiology theory and application to fitness and performance.* 2nd Edition. Dubuque, IA: W.C. Brown Publishing Company, 1994.

U.S. Department of Health and Human Services. *Physical activity and health: A report of the Surgeon General.* Centers for Disease Control and Prevention. National Centers for Chronic Disease Prevention and Health Promotion. Atlanta: The President's Council on Physical Fitness and Sports, 1996.

U.S. Department of Health and Human Services. *Healthy people 2000*: National health promotion and disease prevention objectives. DHHS Publication No (PHS) 91-50213. Washington, D.C.: U.S. Government Printing Office, 1990.

Wilmore, J.H. and D.L. Costill. *Training for sport and activity: The physiological basis of the conditioning process.* 3rd ed. Champaign, IL: Human Kinetics, 1993.

Organizations

American Alliance of Health, Physical Education,
Recreation and Dance (AAHPERD)
1900 Association Drive
Reston, VA 20191-1599
Tel (800) 213-7193
E-mail: info@aahperd.org
Web site: http://www.aahperd.org

American Heart Association
National Center
7272 Greenville Avenue
Dallas, TX 75231
Tel (800) AHA-USA1 (Customer Heart & Stroke
Information)
Tel (888) MY-HEART (Women's Health
Information)
Web site: http://www.aha.org

Videos

Smart Heart: Guide to Cardio-fitness. Explains
cardiovascular system, heart disease and the role of
exercise, nutrition, and stress reduction in
cardiovascular fitness. Cambridge.

How fit are you? YMCA Program Store, Box 5077,
Champaign, IL 61820.

Flexibility

Chapter 4

CHAPTER SUMMARY

You are not likely to die from a lack of flexibility but life with it may more comfortable. Flexibility lets you move more efficiently and aesthetically, enhances sport performance, and helps prevent low-back pain and injury. As you grow older, good flexibility helps retain healthy joint movement which is important to basic living skills.

Many factors influence flexibility, but the most important factor is staying active. Stretching can be part of a warm-up and cool-down, a program of its own, or something you do periodically throughout the day. Stretches are a great way to relieve tension and relax. Static stretches are recommended for general use. Ballistic stretches are recommended only after static stretches and as a means of preparing for vigorous movements. PNF stretching can be used therapeutically or for a general flexibility workout—with a caution that it may cause more muscle soreness. Achieving flexibility and maintaining it can be done at any age, but there are advantages in starting young.

LEARNING OBJECTIVES

The student will be able to:

· explain at least three ways that flexibility can enhance quality of life.
· explain the advantages and disadvantages of static, ballistic, and PNF stretching.
· identify the factors that influence flexibility.
· demonstrate examples of static, ballistic, and PNF stretching.
· demonstrate both active and passive static stretching.
· demonstrate, with proper technique and alignment, a flexibility exercise for each of the major muscles (muscle groups) of the body.
· identify at least three ways to prevent low-back pain.
· determine personal flexibility needs and establish a flexibility plan that will meet those needs.

PERSONAL PROFILE
The Sun City Poms

Their average age is in the 70's and their average kick is well above waist level. Who are these amazing seniors? A group of women in the retirement community of Sun City, Arizona, who formed a dance group to have a little fun and get some exercise. Before long they were performing their dance numbers to enthusiastic audiences and getting national press coverage. What started as an informal local exercise group quickly became a respected traveling performance team called the Sun City Poms.

The Sun City Poms have performed across the United States, appeared before various live audiences, on television, and before the President's Council on Physical Fitness. Their dance numbers range from soft-shoe to pom-poms and include lots of kicks, a few cartwheels and one young member who at the age of seventy steals the show when she drops into the splits.

The group continues to practice and perform regularly because it makes them feel good physically and mentally. They are encouraged to be creative and there are tremendous opportunities to socialize, not only with one another but also with their audience. The Sun City Poms are quick to point out that flexibility and physical activity are not just for the young—this group of seniors has opened many people's eyes to what it means to keep moving for health and enjoyment.

Personal Communication with the Sun City Poms organization, Sun City, Arizona.

CONTENT OUTLINE

I. What exactly is flexibility
    1. flexibility is defined as the range of motion (ROM) around a joint or a group of joints
    2. many joints are multidirectional
    3. you need to maintain full ranges of motion in all directions
II. The anatomy of stretching
    A. an understanding of the muscles, bones, and connective tissues that compose a joint is helpful
    B. in healthy joints, movement is limited to a normal range of motion by the bony structures and connective tissues that make up the joint
        1. connective tissue binds, supports and strengthens other tissues of the joint
            a) elastic connective tissue, like a rubber band, will return to its original shape when it is not being stretched
            b) plastic connective tissue does not have the same ability to retract after stretching
        2. joint capsule, a sack like structure made of tough fibrous connective tissue, surrounds the ends of the bones that make up the joint
    C. synovial fluid in the joint cavity lubricates the cartilage on the ends of the bones
    D. deep fascia, the connective tissue that surrounds and subdivides muscle tissue
        1. the outer layer envelops the whole muscle, and inner layers surround individual muscle fibers and fiber bundles
        2. layers of deep fascia join at the ends of the muscles to form tendons, connective tissue that links the muscle to bone
    F. ligaments are connective tissue that attach one bone to another
        1. ligaments hold bones together in their proper positions
        2. if ligaments are too long, the joint will be looser than it should be, known as joint laxity
            a) injured (overstretched) ligaments and tendons tend to remain somewhat lengthened
                (1) results in a condition of joint instability

            (2) strengthen the muscles around the joint to add stability to the area

    3. to avoid damaging ligaments and tendons during stretching, pay close attention to technique and alignment

    4. most of the flexibility of a joint is determined by the muscles and their fascia

    5. muscle tissue is elastic—sarcomeres (the contractile units that make up muscle fiber) can be stretched to 150 percent of their resting length

        a) to achieve good muscle stretch, the muscle fibers need to be relaxed

        b) as the muscle elongates, the deep fascia will adapt to a stretching program by becoming more resistant to elongation and by increasing their resting length

III. Factors that influence flexibility

  A. Age

    1. erosion of flexibility happens slowly over the years

    2. flexibility increases each year between the ages of 6 and 18

        a) girls more flexible than boys

    3. flexibility increases slow down and stabilize during the late teens and early twenties

  B. Physical activity

    1. flexibility seems to decline with age; the decline largely depends on the individual

        a) sedentary individuals are relatively inflexible

        b) active individuals of all ages tend to maintain or even increase their flexibility

        c) connective tissue does lose some of its elasticity and hydration with age

    2. the secret to healthy, flexible joints is to use them, to move and be active

    3. when muscles are totally immobilized, they can quickly lose range of motion

    4. by identifying which of your muscles are kept in shortened positions, you can concentrate on flexibility exercises for them

  C. Muscle temperature

    1. warm muscles stretch more easily than cold ones

        a) warming up increases blood circulation to the muscles and decreases the viscosity of fluids in the joint capsule and connective tissue

            (1) warming up allows tissues to slide across one another more easily

    2. when you perform flexibility tests, it is important to perform successive tests under the same conditions

        a) make note of the conditions under which you take the test and try to repeat the conditions in subsequent tests

            (1) recommended that flexibility exercises be done after a body-warming experience

  D. Gender

    1. women and girls tend to be more flexible than their male counterparts

        a) influenced to some extent by the nature of activities in which each gender has traditionally participated

  E. Body composition

    1. two instances in which body composition plays a role in flexibility

        a) one is an abundance of adipose tissue

        b) so much muscle bulk that one muscle butts up against another and limits the movement

  F. Disease

        1.   diseases like arthritis can make it uncomfortable or even very painful to move joints

            a)   if you suffer from a joint-affecting disease, consult a physician for suggestions

  G.   Injury

        1.   injury can severely limit range of motion; a good rehabilitation program can help you regain all or a good portion of your flexibility and strength

IV.   Benefits of flexibility

  A.   good flexibility allows for more efficient and effective movement

  B.   relaxation is another benefit of stretching

        1.   it feels good to stretch and bend

  C.   stretching is also helpful for relieving muscle cramps caused by fatigue, overheating, or hormonal changes

        1.   to relieve a cramp, you need to put the contracted muscle into a stretch position

            a)   when you first stretch the muscle, it will be painful, but the cramp will soon dissipate

            b)   massaging the stretching muscle will also help

        2.   stretching after a workout helps relieve and prevent muscle soreness by assisting the fatigued muscles to return to their normal length

V.   Preventing back pain

  A.   one of the best reasons to stay flexible is to prevent back pain

        1.   a large percentage of people (80 percent) experience back pain at some point during their lives

            a)   most cases can be traced to weak abdominal and spinal muscles

            b)   poor muscular endurance

            c)   inadequate flexibility in the spine, hips, and legs

            d)   chronically poor posture

                 (1)   in addition to reducing back pain, good posture makes you look better

        2.   to prevent or relieve back pain, it is helpful to understand the spine and supporting muscles

            a)   three major natural curves, the lumbar, thoracic, and cervical curves

                (1)   back pain is often the result of a reduction in or accentuation of one of these curves

                (2)   lordosis, a condition in which there is excessive curvature in the lower back

            b)   thoracic curve is affected when chest muscles are strengthened more than the back muscles

                (1)   most common among men who want to develop their chest muscles

            c)   poor posture over many years can result in a permanent rounding of the upper spine known as kyphosis

        3.   functional scoliosis occurs when the spine takes on a C or S curve because muscles are shorter on one side of the body

        4.   structural scoliosis which is the result of a structural defect such as incorrect bone formation or a short leg

            a)   functional scoliosis can lead to structural scoliosis if left unchecked

        5.   the cervical curve is most often affected when the jaw or chin is jutted forwarded

        6.   relaxation, posture awareness, proper strength work and the right flexibility exercises can help you maintain a healthy muscle balance along your spine

VI.   Muscle reflexes and flexibility
    A.   Stretch reflex
        1.   nestled in among the muscle fibers are special sensors called muscle spindles
            a)   their job is to keep track of muscle length and the rate (speed) at which muscle length changes
                (1)   when a muscle is stretched, the spindle is stretched and when the spindle is stretched it sends a message to the spinal cord
                    (a)   the more a muscle is stretched or the faster it is stretched the stronger the message
                        (i)   the spinal cord responds with a command to the muscle to contract when the amount or speed of the stretch is thought to endanger the muscle or in the cases of postural muscles, when body position is about to be lost, stretched reflex
        2.   Stretching implications
            a)   muscle spindle activation results in muscle contraction, which hinders the ability of the muscle to stretch
                (1)   the muscle spindle will always react to a lengthening of the muscle fibers
    B.   Inverse myotatic reflex
        1.   another kind of sensor, the Golgi tendon organ (GTO) is located right in the tendon
            a)   GTO's are sensitive to tension
                (1)   tension is created in the tendon both when the muscle stretches and when it contracts
                    (a)   when muscle tension exceeds the GTO's threshold, the GTO sends a signal to the spinal cord
                    (b)   the spinal cord then issues a reflexive message to the muscle, making it relax, tension is decreased
        2.   Stretching implications
            a)   put a muscle into a stretch position, then hold it there long enough, the muscle tension will elicit the inverse myotatic reflex, the muscle will reflectively relax and you will be able to stretch a little further
    C.   Reciprocal innervation
        1.   when one muscle is contracting, the nervous system signals its paired muscle to relax and lengthen
            a)   the nervous system orchestrates the simultaneous increases and decreases in the tensions of the two muscles so well that all we consciously experience is smooth coordinated movement
                (1)   the muscles' complementary responses are called reciprocal innervation
        2.   stretching implications
            a)   during a flexibility exercise, you help relax a muscle by consciously contracting its paired muscle: this is called active stretching
VII.   Methods of stretching

A. there are three types of stretches: static, ballistic, and proprioreceptive neuromuscular facilitation (PNF)

  1. static and ballistic stretches may be performed using either an active or passive stretching technique

  2. PNF, by definition, uses a combination of passive and active stretches

B. Active and Passive stretching

  1. passive stretching occurs when something or someone else creates a stretch in your muscles

    a) because an outside force is helping you stretch, this is often referred to as assisted stretching

    b) a partner creates a passive stretch by moving your muscles into a stretched position and holding you there

      (1) while your partner does the holding, you relax and let the muscle lengthen

  2. active stretch requires contracting one muscle in an effort to stretch another

    a) this works well as long as the contracting muscle is strong enough to pull the other muscle through a full stretch

    b) when you use active stretching, the muscle is said to move through an active range of motion (ROM)

  3. Range of Motion (ROM)

    a) defined as the movement achieved in a joint through self-initiated muscle contraction

    b) passive ROM is the movement of the joint achieved by an outside force such as gravity or a partner

      (1) injuries tend to occur more often in joints that have a larger difference between passive and active ranges of motion

C. Static stretching

  1. to perform a static stretch, move slowly into the stretch position and then hold (without moving) for a minimum of 10 seconds

    a) holding the stretch quiets the stretch reflex and elicits the inverse myotatic reflex

    b) the stretch should be held at a point of discomfort but not pain

      (1) performing a series of static stretches works even better because the GTO's thresholds are reset at a less sensitive level following the first stretch

D. Ballistic stretching

  1. a ballistic stretch is one for which you put the muscle rapidly in and out of stretch position by bouncing or pulsing during the stretch

    a) ballistic stretching will improve flexibility

  2. some significant drawbacks

    a) the rapid lengthening of the muscle elicits the stretch reflex, causing the muscle to contract, the opposite effect desired in a stretch

    b) because the movement is more forceful, it has the potential to injure the muscle and connective tissue

E. PNF stretching

       1.   Proprioceptive neuromuscular facilitation (PNF) stretching was originally developed as a rehabilitation tool

       2.   PNF stretching is the most effective type of stretching

           a)   requires a trustworthy and patient partner, considerably more time and can result in more muscle soreness

       3.   three of the most common ways to perform PNF stretching

           a)   contract-relax (FR)

           b)   contract-relax-antagonist-contract (CRAC)

           c)   slow-reversal-hold-relax (SRHR)

VIII.   Designing your flexibility program.

    A.   Determine your flexibility needs and set goals based on these needs.

       1.   perform flexibility tests

       2.   keep a journal

       3.   ask a coach or fitness specialist about sport-specific stretches

       4.   read a book on stretching

    B.   select exercises that will target your goals

    C.   determine how many repetitions of each exercise you will do

    D.   determine when you will do your flexibility exercises

    E.   warm-up the joint before stretching

IX.   Applying the principles of physical activity.

    A.   The FIT Principle

       1.   Frequency—to improve flexibility

       2.   Intensity—stretch to a point of discomfort, not pain

       3.   Time

           a)   static stretching: 10–60 second holds, 2 to 5 repetitions

           b)   ballistic stretching: 10–60 second bouts, 2 to 5 repetitions

           c)   PNF stretching

    B.   Principles of overload and progression

       1.   flexibility overload is accomplished by stretching muscle further than normal

    C.   Principle of reversibility

       1.   flexibility can be maintained by stretching a minimum of three days a week

    D.   Principle of specificity

       1.   you must select exercises or movements that target the joints you want to stretch

X.   Flexibility Exercises

    A.   When doing stretches that enhance flexibility, use good technique; keeping proper body alignment and isolating the muscle(s) you want to stretch will optimize results and minimize injuries

BEHAVIOR BOOSTS: STAGE-BASED STUDENT ACTIVITIES

Precontemplator

·   Make a note of each time a lack of flexibility either makes something uncomfortable to do or stops you from doing it altogether. At the end of the week, examine your notes: your examples might indicate

that it was difficult to unplug the cord behind the computer, sit cross-legged on the floor, or dip on the dance floor.
- Identify a flexible person and look at the quality of his or her movements. Select an adjective to describe what you see. For example: fluid or relaxed.
- Perform one or more flexibility tests.

Contemplator
- Identify times in your day when you could fit in a flexibility-enhancing movement or exercise.
- Read a book or an article on flexibility.
- Talk to other people about how they stay flexible.
- Find another person interested in enhancing his or her flexibility.
- Take some flexibility tests and decide which areas of flexibility you would most like to improve.
- Choose one exercise and consider adding it to your daily routine.

Preparer
- Experiment with one or more of the flexibility ideas listed under action taker.
- Look for a friend who will join you in a stretching commitment.
- Sign up for a flexibility activity or an activity that includes flexibility exercises, such as yoga, weight training, dance, or one of the martial arts.
- Select one flexibility exercise and set a date for when you will be doing it on a regular basis. (For idea, use the action taker list.)

Action Taker
- After walking up or down stairs, stretch your calves on the top or bottom step. (Be sure to hold on to the a railing.)
- While seated, perform ankle circles and then actively stretch by flexing your ankles.
- After walking outside, stretch your calves on the curb or by leaning against something like a telephone pole.
- Bend forward in your chair (as if to touch the ground) to stretch your low back.
- Change the side your paper is on during typing so your head has to turn the opposite way.
- When your car is stopped at a red light, do some shoulder rolls and shrugs to warm up, then pinch together the shoulder blades. The latter is an active stretch for the chest and shoulder muscles. These exercises can also be done periodically during desk or computer work.
- When standing in a line, touch one foot back with a straight leg and then tuck your pelvis under. This will stretch your hip flexors.
- Place your foot up on a bench, chair, or stair, and lean forward to stretch your hamstring.
- Before going through a doorway, place your hands on either side and lean your chest forward to stretch your shoulder and chest muscles.

Maintainer
- Devise a plan for how to continue flexibility exercises during a business or vacation trip.
- Keep a journal of your activities, exercises, and accomplishments. (Include flexibility test scores over time.)
- Jot down in a journal anything that interrupts your flexibility plan or that tempts you to skip a day.
- Encourage someone else to join you.

ADDITIONAL STUDENT ACTIVITIES

Activity 4.1 Active versus Passive Stretching

Perform the test for active and passive range of motion on text page 82.

LABS

Lab 14.1 What Can I Do? (pages 95–96)
Lab 14.2 Sit-and-Reach Test (page 97)
Lab 14.3 Quick Check Flexibility Tests (pages 98–99)Lab 14.4 Developing Your Flexibility Exercise Program (pages 100–101)

RESOURCES

Suggested Reading

Alter, M.J. *The Science of stretching*. Champaign, IL: Human Kinetics, 1988.

Alter, M.J. *Sports Stretch*. Champaign, IL: Human Kinetics, 1990.

Anderson, B. *Stretching*. Bolinas, CA: Shelter Publications, 1980.

Buroker, K.C., and J.A. Schwane. Does postexercise static stretching alleviate delayed muscle soreness? *The Physician and SportsMedicine* 17(6)65-83, 1989.

Croce, P. *Stretching for athletics*, 2nd ed. Champaign, IL: Leisure Press, 1984.

Gagliardi, N. The joint is jumping: Pain-free workouts. *American Health* 9:36, 1990.

Hardy, L. and D. Jones. Dynamic flexibility and proprioreceptive neuromuscular facilitation. *Research Quarterly for Exercise and Sport* 57:150, 1996.

Kisner, C. and L.A. Colby, *Therapeutic exercises: Foundations and techniques*, Philadelphia: F.A. Davis, 1985.

Kurz, T. *Stretching scientifically: A guide to flexibility training*, 3rd ed. Island Pond, VT: Stadion Publishers, 1994.

McAtee, R.E. *Facilitated stretching*: PNF stretching made easy. Champaign, IL: Human Kinetics, 1993.

Reuler, J.B. Low back pain. *Western Journal of Medicine* 143:259-265, 1985.

Shaw, D.A. Back to back fitness. *Corporate Fitness and Recreation* 2(1):31-37, 1983.

Organizations

American Council on Exercise (ACE)
6190 Cornerstone Court, East, Suite 202
San Diego, CA 92121-4729
5820 Oberlin Drive, Suite 102
San Diego, CA 92121-3787
Tel (619) 535-8227
Fax (619) 535-1778
Web site: http://www.ACEfitness.org

American Heart Association
National Center
7272 Greenville Avenue
Dallas, TX 75231
Tel (800) AHA-USA1 (Customer Heart & Stroke
Information)
Tel (888) MY-HEART (Women's Health
Information)
Web site: http://www.aha.org

Cooper Institute for Aerobic Research (CIAR)
12330 Preston Road
Dallas, TX 75230
Tel (800)-635-7050
Fax (972) 341-3224
Web site: http://www.cooperinst.org

IDEA
6190 Cornerstone Court East, Suite 204
San Diego, CA 92121-3773
Tel (800) 999-4332 ext. 7
Tel (619) 535-8979 ext. 7
Fax (619) 535-8234
Home page: http://www.ideafit.com

Videos

Back Pain How to prevent or lessen severity, how and why pain occurs. Different kinds of problems and treatment. Cambridge Physical Education and Health, P.O. Box 2153, Dept. P.E. 8, Charleston, WV 25328-2153.

Back Safety Video Training Programs, guides and student booklets. Kramer, 1-800-333-3032.

Oh My Aching Back. Commentary by noted orthopaedics; comprehensive, focus on prevention and rehabilitation. Cambridge.

Say Goodbye to Back Pain. Easy to understand explanation of causes of lower back pain, six tests to determine problem areas, tips on pain prevention, and a 3-stage program of exercise. Human Kinetics Publishers.

Muscular Strength and Endurance

Chapter 5

CHAPTER SUMMARY

Muscular strength and endurance are two important health-related components of physical fitness. Improving strength and endurance can be done through traditional weight training methods or using other forms of resistance such as exercise bands, water exercises and even daily activities like washing windows. Good muscle endurance and strength allow you to do more with less fatigue and with less risk of injury. Strength and endurance will also enhance sports performance. There are many types of resistance programs, some emphasizing strength, others endurance, size or power, but most people choose a workout that provides a general fitness emphasis. The latter can be obtained by performing 8–12 repetitions, one to three times each for 8–10 exercises, two or three days a week.

LEARNING OBJECTIVES

Students will be able to:

- define and differentiate between muscular strength and endurance.
- define the terms weight training, resistance training, weight lifting, body building and body sculpting.
- describe the benefits of muscular strength and endurance training.
- explain how muscular strength and endurance relate to daily activities.
- describe the anatomy and physiology of a muscle.
- describe fast twitch and slow twitch fibers and relate them to muscle metabolism.
- describe gender differences concerning absolute and relative strength and hypertrophy.
- identify the major side effects of anabolic steroids.
- differentiate between static and dynamic exercises and give examples of both.
- apply the principles of exercise to muscle strength and endurance.
- differentiate between programs for general fitness, power, hypertrophy, strength, and endurance.
- describe circuit resistance training.
- assess personal strength and endurance.
- identify some of the common errors made when trying to strengthen the abdominal muscles.
- design a personal resistance training program.
- demonstrate a strength/endurance exercise for each of the major muscle groups of the body.

PERSONAL PROFILE

Elle McPherson

The benefits of physical fitness are primarily thought of as being related to health and the prevention of disease. Another benefit of fitness is the change in body shape that occurs when fitness is increased through regular aerobic and strength training exercises. Just ask someone who makes a living because of her body shape. Elle McPherson is the six foot tall model who has graced, among others, the cover of the <u>Sports Illustrated</u> swimsuit issue. As a regular participant in aerobic and strength exercises, Elle enjoys the benefits of having a body that is fit and healthy.

In recent times, the modeling world has changed to reflect the notion that a women can look strong and athletic but still have a woman's curves. To get that look, more and more models are eating more healthfully and participating in resistance-type exercises like lifting weights. Strength training helps Elle and others reduce body fat and increase muscle mass, which results in a firmer, more toned-looking body. Resistance exercises condition and strengthen muscles, resulting in a flatter abdomen, firmer legs and arms, better posture, and increased energy. The general public now seems to prefer this healthier look.

For Elle, it is important to be fit but not fanatic. Three days of strength training a week are enough to maintain muscle strength and good health. In addition to resistance training, she also participates in regular aerobic exercise. By being fit, she has been able to maintain the body which has made her one of the most successful models ever.

Norton, D. Fit but not fanatic: Elle. <u>American Health</u>, 7(6)76-77, 1988.

CONTENT OUTLINE

I.   Health-related muscular strength and endurance
   A.   Wellness requires enough strength and endurance to handle daily activities, leisure activities and emergencies.
   B.   To participate in competitions, athletics or physically challenging leisure activities, you will need a higher level of muscular strength and endurance.
   C.   Muscles get stronger when they work against a greater than normal resistance.
II.   Names for resistance training programs
   A.   Weight training and resistance training
      1.   weight training is used to describe strengthening exercises because weights have been the traditional source of resistance
      2.   resistance training is a newer, more encompassing term than weight training
      3.   muscles can be strengthened using forms of resistance other than weights
         a.   some machines have substituted weight plates with hydraulic or pneumatic pressure, electrical resistance, or thick rubber bands
         b.   pushing and pulling against water in a pool
            (1)   polystyrene dumbbells and webbed gloves can be used to increase resistance
         c.   exercise bands, tubing, and stretch cables
         d.   pressing against an immovable object or against your own body
   B.   Muscular strength training
      1.   is the amount of force that a muscle or muscle group can exert at one time

    2.   basic strength is something many Americans need to improve and maintain

        a.   by age 70 almost one-third of men and two-thirds of women can't pick up as little as ten pounds

            (1)   inactive lifestyle coupled with aging can diminish strength

            (2)   strength gains are maximized by working against a heavy resistance

            (3)   strength is generally practiced using submaximal loads

                (a)   relatively high (not maximum) levels of resistance that can be lifted for a low number of repetitions

C.   Muscular endurance training

    1.   muscular endurance is defined as the ability to:

        a.   exert a submaximal force repeatedly

        b.   maintain a submaximal force for an extended period of time

    2.   the first part describes repetitive muscular contractions, developed using light to moderate resistance for a moderate to high number of repetitions

    3.   the second part describes isometrically held contractions

        a.   contractions in which muscles are exerting force but not moving

        b.   anytime a body position needs to be maintained in a fixed position, isometric contractions are occurring

    4.   often both kinds of muscle endurance are required at the same time

D.   Weight lifting, body building, and body sculpting

    1.   weight lifting and body building are competitive sports

        a.   weight lifting contests involve several types of lifts in which the objective is to lift as much weight as possible each time

        b.   body building is a contest of muscle size, symmetry, and definition

            (1)   winners are able to pose with confidence, showing off their strengths and minimizing their weaknesses

                (a)   train with heavy weights to develop muscle definition

                (b)   use high number of repetitions with lighter weights to develop muscle size

            (2)   gender differences prevent women body builders from achieving the same muscle size increases as men

                (a)   women body building contests stress body proportions and symmetry more than size

        c.   body sculpting is the process of developing a well-proportioned physique

E.   Athletics (sports) and weight training

    1.   athletes in sports other than weight lifting, body building and body sculpting use weight-training programs as a way to improve their motor performance and prevent injury

    2.   performing an advanced program without the proper progressions and a high fitness level can be dangerous

        a.   learn the basic principles and concepts that underlie all resistance training and you will be able to recognize, select and create a program to fit your needs

III.   The strength-endurance continuum

    A.   Muscular strength and endurance are closely related, but distinct components of physical fitness.

        1.   the relationship is defined as a continuum, with maximum strength to the far left and maximum endurance to the far right

            a.   far left activities include weight lifting, football blocking, pushing a car out of a ditch, etc.

            b.   far right activities include marathon running, the Tour de France (cycling), swimming the English Channel, etc.

        2.   in the middle of the continuum there is no clear-cut place where strength leaves off and endurance begins

        3.   the same exercise (or activity) can be a strength workout for one person and a muscular endurance one for someone else

    B.   strength training is often used as a general term to describe both strength and endurance exercises

IV.   Muscle anatomy and physiology

    A.   How muscles work

        1.   the connective tissue surrounding the center (belly) of a muscle tapers off to form one or more muscle tendons at each end

            a.   the tendons attach to bones on opposite sides of a joint

                (1)   when the muscle contracts, its tendon(s) are pulled in toward the belly of the muscle bringing the attached bone(s) with them

        2.   Fitness implications

        3.   to achieve good body symmetry, opposing muscles should both be exercised

            a.   imbalances can result in injury, loss of flexibility, or poor posture

    B.   Muscle fibers

        1.   inside the connective tissue, each muscle is made up of bundles of muscle fibers (cells)

            a.   these bundles, called fasciculi (or fascicles), give the muscle form and structure

                (1)   the fibers inside the fasciculi are arranged in different ways according to the function of the muscle

                    (a)   muscles that need to move bones through wide ranges of motion have fasciculi with fibers running longitudinally

                        i)   this allows for maximum contraction (contracting to about one-half its length)

                    (b)   the longer the fibers, the greater the contraction and resulting movement of the bone

                (2)   other muscles have fasciculi with fibers running diagonally

                    (a)   these fibers are shorter but also more plentiful

                    (b)   the more plentiful but shorter the fibers in a muscle, the greater the capacity for strength with a more limited range of motion

            b.   each fiber is made up of smaller strands called myofibrils

             c.   myofibrils are made up of even smaller protein strands called myofilaments

                (1)   there are two kinds of myofilaments: the thicker myosin and the thinner actin

            d.   the myosin and the actin myofilaments are arranged in units called sarcomeres

                (1)   these line up end to end to make up the myofibril

                (a)   the sarcomere segments are what give skeletal muscle a striated appearance

          (2)   sliding filament theory—sarcomeres contract when the myosin and actin fibers slide over one another

2.   fitness implications

    a.   resistance training, which is primarily anaerobic, increases the amount of energy, ATP and PC that can be stored directly in the muscle fiber

          (1)   this energy can then be used to fuel contractions

    b.   the muscle's tolerance to lactic acid increases

          (1)   can perform more work (contractions) before experiencing exhaustion

C.   The motor unit

    1.   is made up of one motor neuron and the fiber(s) it innervates

        a.   to move a muscle, a message is sent from the brain (or spinal cord) to the muscles via nerve fibers called motor neurons

            (1)   small motor units (one motor neuron innervating only a small number of fibers) are necessary for precise, delicate work, such as that performed by the eye muscles

            (2)   large motor units (one motor neuron innervating a large number of fibers) are found in muscles used for heavy work loads

        b.   when a motor unit contracts, all of the fibers in the unit contract

        c.   the strength of a contraction is orchestrated by recruiting the correct number and type of fibers

    2.   fitness implications

        a.   strategies for maximizing fiber recruitment have been devised to develop the muscle more fully

            (1)   if you fatigue the initially recruited fibers, additional fibers will be recruited

                 (a)   this occurs when you perform (1) a high number of consecutive repetitions (2) more than one set of repetitions (3) two exercises in a row that work the same muscle

D.   Slow twitch and fast twitch fibers

    1.   muscle fibers are made up of different kinds of fibers with different metabolic roles

        a.   slow twitch fibers (ST) work best under aerobic conditions and are often referred to as Type I, red, or slow oxidative (SO) fibers

            (1)   slow twitch fibers contract more slowly and are capable of sustaining low to moderate intense contractions over much longer periods of time

        b.   fast twitch, Type II, white, and fast-glycolytic (FG) fibers are named because they have greater speed and contractility.

            (1)   used for explosive anaerobic movements like sprinting and a badminton smash

            (2)   are rich in stored energy, can react quickly, but for only a short time

            (3)   there are two types of fast twitch fibers

                 (a)   FTa (Type IIa) fibers possess some of the oxidative (aerobic) properties of ST fibers and some of the anaerobic properties of FTb

            (b)   FTb (Type IIb) have higher concentrations of stored phosphocreatine (PC) and glycogen

    2.   ST, FTa, and FTb, all have some aerobic and anaerobic capability

       a.   FTa is somewhere in the middle, and FTb has the least aerobic but most anaerobic capabilities

       b.   all the fibers in one motor unit are the same type, but within muscles they can be motor units of different types

           (1)   percentages of FTa, FTb and ST vary from person to person and to some extent from muscle to muscle on one person

       c.   a muscle biopsy can determine a person's percentages of fast and slow twitch fibers

    3.   fitness implications

       a.   aerobic and muscular endurance conditioning will improve the ability of ST and FTa fibers to generate and use energy

       b.   speed and strength conditioning will enhance FT fibers

E.   Muscle fuels

    1.   fuel source for muscle contraction varies with the intensity and volume of the program

       a.   very intense, short exercise bouts (1 to 30 seconds) depend on the stored energy available through the ATP-PC system

           (1)   this system can be trained through a resistance program that emphasizes strength and power

       b.   lactic acid system becomes the major source of energy for movements that last between 30 seconds and 3 minutes

           (1)   this carbohydrate-burning system produces ATP for energy with a simultaneous buildup of lactic acid

    2.   fitness implications

       a.   training regimens that use a moderate to high intensity and a few to moderate number of repetitions trains the lactic acid system

       b.   high-number repetitions, low-resistance exercises draw energy from both the lactic acid system and aerobic glycolysis

       c.   resistance training is not a substitute for aerobic training for increasing aerobic capacity

V.   Gender differences

A.   Absolute and relative strength

    1.   regardless of the gender, muscle tissue creates a force of 3 to 8 kilograms per square centimeter of cross section

       a.   more of a man's weight is attributable to muscle

       b.   men have a higher percentage of their muscle in their upper body as compared to the lower body

    2.   absolute strength refers to the actual amount of weight or resistance a person handles

    3.   relative strength compares two people's strength with an adjustment made for differences in muscle mass

B.   Hypertrophy and strength

    1.   an increase in muscle size is called hypertrophy

2.   a decrease in muscle size is called atrophy
3.   hypertrophy is the result of an increase in fiber size and not an increase in the number of fibers
       a.   men and women hypertrophy at the same rate
       b.   women's muscle fibers are smaller than men's, therefore men's muscles tend to be bigger
            (1)   body composition changes can cause circumference measures to be misleading
               (a)   women have more fat between muscle fibers than men

C.   Transient hypertrophy
    1.   is a temporary muscle enlargement following resistance training
    2.   caused by an accumulation of water in the muscle
       a.   resistance exercise temporarily upsets a homeostatic state, resulting in an accumulation of fluid (mostly water) in the interstitial and cellular spaces of the muscle
            (1)   this condition, called edema, causes the muscle to be larger than normal
            (2)   women's muscles are smaller so the hypertrophy is less apparent

D.   Training implications
    1.   women respond to the same training program as well as or better than men
    2.   resistance training provides additional benefits for women who carry and deliver a child
       a.   strong muscles help pregnant women maintain good posture, and handle extra weight

VI.   The effects of anabolic steroids on muscles
    A.   anabolic steroid pills and injections, synthetic versions of the male hormone testosterone, can increase muscle strength and growth, but also have dangerous side effects including death (see text page 113)
    B.   human growth hormones (HGH) are also used to promote muscle and bone growth and heal tendons and ligaments
    C.   when the natural growth rate is accelerated in this way, there is tremendous opportunity for long-range irreversible problems
    D.   are illegal unless prescribed by a physician

VII.   static and dynamic training
    A.   two types of exercises for muscles: static and dynamic
    B.   static exercise is performed without movement
    C.   dynamic exercises are the opposite; they involve movements through a range of motion
    D.   strength gains tend to be specific to the type of training the muscle receives
       1.   for dynamic strength, it is best to train dynamically
       2.   for static strength, train statically
          a.   static strength is important for postural muscles, and static strength exercises are important in rehabilitation
          b.   static strength may be achieved using isometric contractions (exercises)
            (1)   in isometric contraction, the muscle fibers contract, but the length of the muscle does not change

   c. dynamic strength can be developed using either isotonic or isokinetic contractions (exercises)

     (1) an isotonic contraction is one in which the tension in the muscle stays the same throughout the range of motion

  3. weight training equipment, universal, and nautilus machines are called "variable resistance" machines

  4. free weights (barbells and dumbbells) provide a constant resistance and have therefore been named "constant resistance" or "fixed resistance" exercises

  5. it is technically incorrect to call both constant and variable resistance training isotonic training

 E. dynamic contractions can be described according to the lengthening or shortening of the muscle fibers

  1. when the muscle is shortening, it is said to be concentric contraction

  2. when the muscle is lengthening, it is said to be eccentric contraction

   a. sometimes concentric contractions are referred to as positives

   b. eccentric contractions are referred to as negatives

     (1) negatives can be performed using heavier loads than positives, because you are slowing the weight's descent as opposed to pushing it up against gravity

   c. eccentric weight training requires one or more partners to help raise the weight to a starting position

 F. isokinetic contractions exert force through a range of motion at a designated speed

 G. isokinetic and variable resistance exercises can more effectively challenge the strong points in the strength curve

  1. they are no more effective than fixed resistance exercises in their ability to strengthen the weak point

VIII. Applying the principles of physical activity

 D. FIT Principle

  1. frequency

   a. resistance training performed two to three times a week with a 48-hour rest between workouts is recommended for moderate improvements in strength and endurance

     (1) twice a week is minimum for developing strength

     (2) once a week may maintain strength if the workout is performed at the same intensity you trained at to achieve the strength

  2. intensity

   a. to emphasize strength, intensity is increased by adding resistance and maintaining or lowering repetitions

   b. to emphasize endurance, the resistance is increased but is done more gradually in order to continue using a high number of repetitions

  3. time

   a. the length of the workout is influenced by the number of repetitions of an exercise and the number of sets of repetitions performed

     (1) the number of repetitions falls between one and twenty and the number of sets falls between one and five

> > > (a)   between each set is a rest break (10 to 30 seconds) used to develop endurance
> > > (b)   rest breaks of 1 to 3 minutes allow for greater recovery and are used to space strength exercises that require more of a maximal effort

> > 4.   mode
> > > a.   activities such as tennis, golf, and washing the car can help build and maintain muscular endurance
> > > b.   strength is built through calisthenics or activities that are challenging enough that you can do only about six to ten repetitions or through a resistance training program like weight training

> E.   Principles of progression and overload (progressive overload)
> > 1.   increase the load (weight) in dynamic exercises
> > 2.   increase the force exerted against an immovable object in isometric exercises
> > 3.   increase the force exerted through a range of motion in isokinetic exercises
> > 4.   shorter rest breaks between sets also increases overload

> F.   Principle of specificity
> > 1.   exercise technique and form ensure that the target muscle is exercised
> > > a.   if muscles other than the targeted muscle (or muscle group) are allowed to be used during an exercise, less training of the targeted muscle occurs

> G.   Principle of reversibility
> > 1.   when muscles are challenged they get stronger; when muscles are inactive or face less rigorous activity than normal they grow weaker

> H.   Principle of individuality
> > 1.   the rate and potential to which you will develop strength and endurance will naturally be different from someone else's
> > 2.   different programs work for different people
> > 3.   individualize your program and try not to judge your progress against others

IX.   Manipulating resistance training program variables
> A.   Strength program
> > 1.   dynamic strength
> > > a.   the greatest amount of weight (load) that a person can lift, push or pull at one time is referred to as one repetition max or 1 RM
> > > > (1)   one to six repetitions are performed to the point of voluntary exhaustion
> > > > > (a)   you use a weight that you can lift six times, but not seven; this is referred to as one set of 6 RM
> > > > (2)   multiple sets (two to five) are recommended for optimal strength gains
> > > b.   a program that emphasizes strength uses and develops the ATP-PC and lactic acid energy systems
> > > > (1)   breaks should be 2 to 3 minutes between sets
> > > > > (a)   the ATP-PC system can produce energy very quickly for short bouts (1 to 3 seconds) of exercise, but once used takes several minutes to recover

           (2)   different sets can use the same resistance or be of increasing or decreasing amounts of resistance

2.   Isometric strength

    a.   isometric strength training is particularly helpful for developing strength in one position

        (1)   isometric contractions of maximal force held for duration of 30 seconds will result in strength gains

        (2)   strength gain is limited to the joint angle used in the exercise and a carryover of about 20 degrees in both directions

        (3)   advantages

            (a)   little or no equipment required

            (b)   exercises can be performed alone or with an exercise partner

            (c)   can be helpful in getting past the sticking point in dynamic exercise

            (d)   stabilizing strength can be developed for one position

3.   Muscular endurance program

    a.   developed using lighter weights for a high number of repetitions

        (1)   no upper limit on the number of repetitions

            (a)   strength training also increases endurance; therefore, limiting the number to ten to twenty may be a more efficient use of time

4.   General fitness program

    a.   ACSM recommends the average healthy adult perform a minimum of eight to ten resistance training exercises involving the major muscle groups, a minimum of twice a week.

    b.   a minimum of one set of eight to twelve repetitions to near fatigue should be completed for each exercise

5.   Power program

    a.   achieved by manipulating the amount of the resistance and the speed with which it is moved

    b.   power is often equated with strength, but it is a combination of strength and speed

    c.   power training can be strength-related or speed-related and the combination program varies depending upon the desired outcome

6.   Hypertrophy program

    a.   train in a way that causes one set of muscle fibers to become fatigued so that additional fibers are recruited

        (1)   high volume of sets and repetitions

            (a)   multiple sets (two to five) of eight to fifteen repetitions are generally recommended

                i)   lactic acid system is the major supplier of energy

                ii)   primarily FT fibers are recruited

7.   Circuit resistance training program

    a.   circuit training means to move from one exercise into the next with little or no break between exercises

          (1)   can be designed for muscular strength and endurance or cardiorespiratory endurance or a combination of the two

          (2)   circuit resistance training (CRT) emphasizes muscular endurance and may provide some aerobic benefit

                 (a)   not a substitute for aerobic exercise

          (3)   distinct advantages

                 (a)   if using machines, relatively quick and easy

                 (b)   takes about one minute per station to set the weight, get into position and perform the repetitions, which means twelve-exercise circuits can be done in fifteen minutes

          (4)   circuit training can also be done with free weights

          (5)   mini-circuits consisting of three or four exercises can also be performed

X.   Designing a resistance exercise program

    A.   Assess your needs

        1.   assess your present level of strength and endurance for the major muscles

        2.   think about the types of activities you like to do and determine which muscles are involved and whether the contractions are static or dynamic

    B.   Select your exercises

        1.   based on your general goals, decide which muscles you need to work and select exercises that target them

        2.   organize your selected exercises onto a log sheet

        3.   large-muscle/small-muscle system—large muscles precede small muscles

        4.   upper body/lower body—upper body exercises are alternated with lower-body exercises, an arrangement that ensures a muscle will get a substantial break before being used again

        5.   circuit resistance training (CRT)

    C.   Decide where on the continuum you wish to work

        1.   muscular strength

        2.   general fitness

        3.   muscular endurance

    D.   Determine and record on the log sheet the:

        1.   number of repetitions

        2.   number of sets

        3.   length of breaks

    E.   Determine the frequency of your workouts and record on your selected exercise list which days you will train.

    F.   Determine your resistance for each exercise and record it on your exercise log sheet.

    G.   Set more specific goals.

    H.   Start your program.

BEHAVIOR BOOSTS: STAGE-BASED STUDENT ACTIVITIES

A regular resistance training program is the most effective way to build strength but when that is not possible, or is not of interest, some of these other ideas can help you develop or maintain some muscle tone.

Precontemplator
- List the things you'd like to change about your body. Look at the list to see if any of the changes can be made through resistance activities.
- Examples: I wish my back didn't ache at the end of the day. I've achieved a good body weight, but I wish I felt "firm" instead of "loose."
- Ask people who have a physique you admire how they achieved and maintain it.
- Any time you try to do something and find yourself to be "too weak" jot it down in a notebook. Also include activities that cause you to be very stiff and sore or even cause injury. Review this list at the end of one or two weeks and ask yourself if resistance activities could improve your quality of life.
- Look in a full-length mirror at your posture. Would strengthening and stretching exercises improve it?
- List the sports or leisure time activities you do, or would like to do. Look at this list to determine whether muscular strength and endurance would help you perform better.

Contemplator
- Find and tour the recreational facilities on campus or a club nearby. (Some dormitories also have equipment.)
- If you play sports, determine which muscles should be targeted in your workout.
- Look at the courses offered on resistance training (college, university or recreational courses) and consider whether you would like to sign up for one.

Preparer
- Put together an eight to twelve exercise program.
- If you are going to use homemade equipment, assemble the things you need and create a workout space.
- Sign up for a course or find someone who can teach you how to do resistance exercises properly. Find a workout partner or spotter if you intend to lift free weights.
- Set a start date.

Action Taker
- Do toe raises when waiting in a line or—if you can coordinate it—while brushing your teeth.
- Climb the stairs two at a time.
- Lie on your back and bench press your baby/child or your anatomy and physiology books.
- Arm wrestle.
- Put an exercise band or dumbbells near the television, phone or other place where you tend to sit and talk and use them.
- While seated draw a knee up to your chest, lower, and repeat.
- Pull your shoulder blades together and hold for three to six seconds when in the car and stopped at a light, or periodically during desk or computer work, or after bending over a project such as working on a car engine.
- Put a "stress ball" or hand-grip strengthening device by the phone, on your desk, or in your knapsack and squeeze it whenever you are angry or fidgety.

- Press against the ceiling of the car with both arms when you are stopped at a light, stuck in traffic, or anytime as a passenger. (Because this is an isometric contraction people with high blood pressure should first check with their physicians.)
- Purposely carry extra books in your knapsack or bag.
- Alternate the shoulder or arm used to carry bags, parcels, equipment, or children.
- Perform a set of shoulder shrugs as you trek across campus.
- Kick a ball with a friend. Use a variety of kicks, including instep and toe-down kicks and use both legs.

Maintainer
- Invite a friend or family member to join you in your strength and endurance activity.
- Keep a record of your work outs and celebrate improvements.
- Vary your activity to prevent staleness.
- Examples: If you are using weights, try a new system like pyramiding. If you've been climbing steps at home, take a trip to a stadium and climb in the outdoors, or ride a mountain bike up and down hills.
- Plan a special event that takes advantage of your level of strength or endurance.
- Examples: Take a canoe trip. Try a ropes course. Paint the house, put in a fence, and so forth. Pull a child in a wagon on a hilly terrain.

ADDITIONAL STUDENT ACTIVITIES

Activity 5.1: Sample Isometric Exercises

Try the isometric exercises described on text page 114. Think about when and if any of these exercises could fit into your day.

LABS

Lab 5.1 What Can I Do? (pages 141–142)
Lab 5.2 Curl-Up Test (page 143)
Lab 5.3 Push-Up Test (page 144)
Lab 5.4 Weight Training-Muscular Endurance Test (pages 145–146)
Lab 5.5 Developing Your Strength and Endurance Program (pages 147–148)

RESOURCES

Suggested Reading

American College of Sports Medicine. The recommended quantity and quality of exercise for developing and maintaining cardiorespiratory and muscular fitness in healthy adults. *Medicine and Science in Sports* 22(2):265-274, 1990.

Baechle, T.R. and B.R. Groves. *Weight training steps to success*. Champaign, IL: Leisure Press, 1992.

Bartels, R.L. Weight training. *The Physician and Sportsmedicine* 20:233-234, 1992.

Bucci, L.R. *Nutrients as Ergogenic Aids for Sports and Exercise*. Boca Raton, FL: CRC Press, 1993.

The best workout: Free weights vs. machines, *University of California Berkeley Wellness Letter* 9:6, 1993.

Bodybuilding for the nineties, *Nutrition Action Health Letter* 19:1, 5-7, 1992.

Fleck, S.J. and W.J. Kraemer. *Designing resistance training programs*, 2nd ed. Champaign, IL: Human Kinetics, 1997.

Gettman, L.R. and M.L. Pollock. Circuit weight training: A critical review of its physiological benefits. *The Physician and Sportsmedicine* 9:44-60, 1981.

Lockette, K.F. and A.M. Keyes. *Conditioning with physical disabilities*. Champaign, IL: Human Kinetics, 1994.

Miller, P.D., ed. *Fitness programming and physical disability*. Champaign, IL: Human Kinetics, 1995.

Strength training, *Mayo Clinic Health Letter* 8:2-3, 1990.
Wilmore, J.H. and D.L. Costill. *Training for sport and activity: The physiological basis of the conditioning process*, 3rd ed. Champaign, IL: Human Kinetics, 1993.

Organizations

American Alliance of Health, Physical Education.
Recreation and Dance (AAHPERD)
1900 Association Drive
Reston, VA 20191-1599
Tel (800) 213-7193
E-mail: info@aahperd.org
Web site: http://www.aahperd.org

American College of Sports Medicine (ACSM)
P.O. Box 1440
Indianapolis, IN 46206-1440
Tel (317) 637-9200
Fax (317) 634-7817
Web site: http://www.acsm.org

The Physician and Sportsmedicine
Web site: www.physsportsmed.com

Striving for Wellness with Proper Nutrition

Chapter 6

CHAPTER SUMMARY

Ideal nutrition is clearly related to good health and reduced disease; unfortunately, the overall quality of the typical American diet is far from ideal. Taste preferences and tradition are but a few reasons why the typical daily consumption of fats and simple sugars is too high and that of fruits and vegetables is too low. Some individuals also struggle to get the proper amounts of calcium, iron, and sodium. Although research continues to refine our knowledge of proper nutrition, consumers should be cautious when making food and supplement selections based on claims of big benefits. Sound advice would be to use the food pyramid as a guide for healthy eating. This chapter reviews the function and sources of the six basic nutrients.

LEARNING OBJECTIVES

The student will be able to:
- identify factors that influence what people eat
- explain the relationship between diet and disease
- name the six basic nutrients and describe their functions
- differentiate between nutrient dense foods and empty calories
- describe the food pyramid and give examples of each type of food
- explain the differences between, and sources of, saturated, monounsaturated and polyunsaturated fats
- list sources of dietary fat common in a college student's diet
- explain the differences between, and sources of, simple and complex carbohydrates
- explain the importance of reducing sugar intake
- identify sources of fiber and explain the roles of soluble and insoluble fiber
- explain the difference between essential and nonessential amino acids
- name three types of vegetarians
- explain the importance of eating fruits and vegetables both for health and in the battle against disease
- identify water-soluble and fat-soluble vitamins
- identify valid reasons for vitamin and mineral supplementation
- explain the role of vitamins in disease prevention
- suggest ways to include sufficient iron and calcium in the diet
- suggest ways to cut down on sodium consumption
- explain what osteoporosis is and how to prevent it
- identify healthy and unhealthy trends in eating

- read and understand a food label
- discuss diet concerns for athletes
- explain the role of exercise in conjunction with nutrition
- select and organize foods into a menu that describes a balanced diet
- initiate a diet change and strive toward maintaining a balanced diet

PERSONAL PROFILE: The College Diet Dilemma

Note: This profile touches on issues involving nutrition (chapter 6), body composition (chapter 7) and weight control (chapter 8). A second profile describing Oprah Winfrey's battle with weight control through nutrition and exercise is available with the chapter 8 instructor manual materials.

My name is Kevin Anderson. I'm a 22-year-old college sophomore majoring in business management. After graduation from high school I started working for a local company as a sales representative. Most of my time was spent traveling by car as I worked to bring in new accounts for my employer. As a high school student I was never an outstanding athlete, but I did play a lot of intramural sports and liked to mountain bike. All that changed when I started working full time. All regular physical activity ceased and my diet was shameful. As a result, my weight went from 176 pounds to 194 pounds in a two-year period and I had 28 percent body fat. That's only slightly less than obese! I wasn't particularly happy with my job and I was depressed with the condition of my body, so I returned to college in hopes of eventually getting better employment and gaining control over my unhealthy lifestyle.

The wellness program at my college was a tremendous help in showing me what I needed to do. They did a fitness assessment to measure my body fat, fitness level, and diet. With the help of one of their health professionals, I started a daily jogging program. My jogging was barely faster than walking, and it was difficult. For the first week, I could only run for about ten minutes, and even then I felt exhausted. By week three, I was able to run for thirty minutes and didn't have to stop to catch my breath.

My battle with weight began to be more effective when I finally changed my diet. I'm embarrassed to say that I used to eat nothing but fast food packed with fat. I did, however, think about the foods I was eating. If I thought it tasted good, I ate it.

I'm a changed person. I have greatly reduced the amount of fat in my diet. Planning ahead for meals, reading labels, buying fruits and vegetables, and carefully selecting fast foods have made a big difference in how I feel and how much I weigh. After four months, I had lost eighteen pounds. I followed this up with twelve more months of regular, moderate exercise and healthy eating and I still haven't gained a pound. I look good, and more important, I feel great. In fact, these feelings of wellness are what keep me committed to my new lifestyle. Even better than feeling trim, I feel like I'm back in control of my life.

CONTENT OUTLINE

I. Introduction
    A. Never before in fitness and wellness has there been more emphasis on the importance of proper nutrition.
    B. Primary sources of nutritional information come from the media mainly in the form of advertisements. Food producers promote benefits, but don't necessarily explain all aspects of their products.

    C.   Optimal nutrition is defined as having a diet that contains enough nutrients for tissue repair, maintenance, and growth without an excess of energy intake.

II.   Food choices are influenced by a number of factors.
    A.   Time of day
    B.   Cost of food
    C.   Religious beliefs
    D.   What our parents eat
    E.   What food looks like
    F.   A busy schedule

III.   Our choice of foods affects our health.
    A.   Convenience foods tend to be high in fat, sodium, etc.
    B.   Nutritional deficiency in the U.S. is rare; however, 6 out of the 10 leading causes of death are associated with what we eat.
    C.   Coronary heart disease, stroke, cancer, diabetes, arteriosclerosis and liver disease are not related to nutritional deficiencies; they can be caused by poor food choices or by overeating.
    D.   Approximately 35 percent of the adult population in the industrialized world is obese, and current estimates indicate that 50 percent of adults in the U.S. are overweight.

IV.   The U.S. Department of Agriculture introduced the food pyramid to improve the quality of our diets.
    A.   The food pyramid, starting at the base (level 1), includes the following six food groups:
        1.   Level 1: Bread, cereal, rice, & pasta group, 6–11 servings
        2.   Level 2: Vegetable group, 3–5 servings
        3.   Level 2: Fruit group, 2–4 servings
        4.   Level 3: Milk, yogurt, & cheese group, 2–3 servings
        5.   Level 3: Meat, poultry, fish, dry beans, eggs, & nuts group, 2–3 servings
        6.   Level 4: Fats, oils and sweets, consume only in the smallest quantity
    B.   To achieve a balanced nutritious diet, one must eat a variety of foods from each food group.

V.   Nutritional standards for vitamins and minerals are known as recommended dietary allowances (RDAs).

VI.   Nutrients are the constituents of food that sustain us physiologically.
    A.   There are six different nutrients found in food.
        1.   fats
        2.   carbohydrates
        3.   protein
        4.   water
        5.   vitamins
        6.   minerals
    B.   A deficiency in any of the nutrients will impair body function.
    C.   Fats, carbohydrates, and protein are sources of energy for the body's physiological processes.
    D.   A kilocalorie, commonly called a calorie, is the standard unit of measure used when referring to the amount of energy a food contains.
        1.   One gram of fat contains nine calories of energy.
        2.   One gram of carbohydrate contains four calories of energy.
        3.   One gram of protein contains four calories of energy.
    E.   Foods with little nutritional value are said to supply "empty calories."
    F.   A balanced diet should contain:

1. no more than 30 % fat
2. 58–60 % carbohydrates (48% complex, 10% simple)
3. 10–12 % protein

VII. Fats
    A. Fat is a necessary component of proper nutrition because it:
        1. helps to insulate and protect vital organs and tissues
        2. provides storage for several fat-soluble vitamins
        3. is an efficient storehouse of energy
    B. Diets high in fat are linked to a number of diseases and conditions including:
        1. obesity
        2. hypertension
        3. stroke
        4. high blood cholesterol
        5. cancer
        6. non-insulin diabetes
        7. heart disease
    C. There is a close relationship between the amount of fat people consume and the amount of body fat they possess.
        1. dietary fat takes less energy to store than carbohydrate (3 calories as compared to 23–27 to store 100 calories of fat and carbohydrate, respectively)
    D. Fats are compounds made by combining fatty acid and glycerol to form glyceride.
        1. Triglycerides have 3 fatty acids attached to one glycerol.
        2. Triglycerides are classified according to the number of chemical bonds they have with hydrogen. Types of triglycerides:
            a. saturated (has all the hydrogen atoms it can hold)
            b. monounsaturated (has room for one more hydrogen atom)
            c. polyunsaturated (has room for more than one hydrogen atom)
        3. Other types of fat include
            a. phospholipids
            b. sterols
    E. Saturated fats
        1. tend to be stable (don't spoil easily)
        2. are usually solids at room temperature
        3. are directly related to elevated blood cholesterol, stroke, coronary heart disease
        4. are used by the liver to produce cholesterol when dietary cholesterol is cut.
            a. For this reason the amount of cholesterol in the bloodstream is thought to be more closely related to the amount of saturated fat in one's diet than to the amount of cholesterol consumed.
        5. taste good, used as thickeners
        6. come from animal products including red meat, cheese, whole milk, butter and cream
        7. also found in coconut and palm oil
        8. average diet consumes 15 % of calories in saturated fat; recommended diet has no more than 10% of its calories from saturated fat
    F. Polyunsaturated and monounsaturated fats
        1. are found in vegetable oils like safflower, olive, and sunflower oil

    2.   average person consumes too much monounsaturated oil and too little polyunsaturated oil

    3.   may help reduce blood cholesterol

G.   Fat substitutes are being used in foods to retain texture and taste but reduce fat content. Long term studies have not been completed on such products.

H.   Fat in a product can be labeled as a percentage of weight or percentage of calories.

    1.   Meat that is 95% fat free by weight can have a high percentage of calories from fat.

    2.   Two percent milk is 2 % fat by weight but 32% of its calories come from fat.

I.   There are a number of ways to reduce fat in the diet.

    1.   limit fried foods, especially those fried in animal, palm or coconut oil

    2.   avoid greasy food

    3.   use lean cuts of meat, trim the fat, skin chicken and turkey

    4.   drink fortified skim milk and eat low-fat cheeses

    5.   use seasonings/herbs in place of high fat gravies and sauces

    6.   limit egg yolk consumption to four a week

    7.   limit red meat, eat more fish

VIII. Carbohydrates

A.   At least 58 % of total daily caloric intake should be carbohydrates

B.   The primary source of energy for all human metabolism

    1.   a shortage of carbohydrates will result in metabolism of fat and protein for energy, which will result in decreased muscle mass and body fat

    2.   are necessary for the body to burn fat

C.   Types:

    1.   simple

    2.   complex

    3.   fiber

D.   Simple Carbohydrates

    1.   are made up of one or two simple sugar molecules

        a.   monosaccharides: glucose, fructose, galactose

        b.   disaccharides: table sugar (glucose + fructose)

    2.   foods containing them (sugars) taste good and are therefore often overeaten

        a.   The average person consumes two and a half times the recommended daily intake of simple sugars.

        b.   The typical American consumes 130 pounds of refined sugar each year.

    3.   Naturally occurring sugars are found in fruits, vegetables, honey and milk.

        a.   Foods low in calories and high in nutrients are considered nutrient dense.

        b.   All fruits and vegetables are nutrient dense.

    4.   Foods made of refined sugars are generally lacking in nutrients and are therefore considered to supply "empty calories."

        a.   Empty calories are a poor source of energy.

        b.   Foods with refined sugars typically do not contain essential vitamins and minerals. Without sufficient vitamins and minerals the body is not able to use available stores of energy.

        c.   Even if a person eats sufficient calories by consuming simple carbohydrates, a deficiency in vitamins or minerals will prevent the body from functioning properly

5. Refined sugars used in packaged foods include high-fructose syrup, honey, sucrose, corn syrup, cornstarch, dextrose, sorghum, and maltose.
6. Methods to reduce sugar in the diet:
    a. Replace soda with unsweetened fruit juices or water.
    b. Gradually reduce the sugar you add to beverages and cereals.
    c. Cut back on the amount of sugar you use in recipes.
    d. Read food labels and cut back on foods that list any type of sugar as one of the first three ingredients.
    e. Buy fruit canned in its own juice rather than in sweetened juices or syrup.
    f. Buy cereals low in sugar and don't add any to them.
    g. Cut back on other major sources of sugar, e.g., pastries, cookies, cakes.
7. Sugar substitutes mimic the chemical structure of sugars in such a way that taste buds tell us they taste sweet.
    a. Sugar-free foods have helped diabetics immensely.
    b. Sugar substitutes include: Nutrasweet, Equal, saccharin, cyclamate

E. Complex Carbohydrates
1. simple sugars that have been connected to form long complex chains
2. often referred to as starches
3. come from plant sources and are therefore often low in calories but high in nutrients
4. food sources include fruits and vegetables
5. diets rich in fruits and vegetables, particularly cruciferous vegetables such as broccoli and cauliflower, offer protection against some forms of cancer
    a. cruciferous vegetables are a good source of antioxidants (substances that inhibit reactions promoted by oxygen)
6. a healthy diet should include 45 percent of its calories from complex carbohydrates
    a. decreases risk of cardiovascular disease, obesity, cancer, and diabetes and may promote fewer cavities
    b. the average person needs to almost double his/her consumption of complex carbohydrates
7. are too often eaten with fattening sauces (e.g., on pasta) or toppings (e.g., sour cream, butter, and chili on potatoes)
8. a diet rich in fruits and vegetables will lower fat intake and increase fiber intake

F. Fiber—a form of complex carbohydrate
1. some experts think fiber should be classified as a seventh basic nutrient
2. often called roughage
    a. humans, unlike many animals, lack the enzymes and bacteria needed to break it down into usable nutrients
3. The National Cancer Institute recommends that we eat 20–35 grams of fiber daily.
    a. the average American consumes less than half of the recommended amount
    b. dietary fiber should be gradually increased over several weeks to prevent gastrointestinal upset
4. two types of fiber are found in every plant food:
    a. soluble
    b. insoluble

     5.   Soluble Fiber
- a. fiber that dissolves in water
- b. Eating soluble fibers like bran and oatmeal, and possibly other high fiber foods like strawberries and brussels sprouts can lower blood cholesterol.
- c. Other good sources include: corn bran, apples, pears, prunes, oranges, sweet potatoes, dried beans, and other fruits, vegetables and legumes. Also gels and pectins.
- d. Gels and pectins dissolve and thicken adding bulk to stomach contents and slowing stomach emptying. This gives a sense of fullness which may help individuals control their eating. Also helps diabetics by slowing the absorption of sugars from the small intestine, lowering insulin requirements and lowering elevated blood pressure.

     6.   Insoluble Fiber
- a. the part of food we consume that is not digested
- b. aids bulk to the intestinal contents, which increases the speed with which food moves through the intestines and produces a softer stool
  - (1) constipation is prevented
  - (2) bulk prevents intestinal contents from becoming compacted, which helps prevent obstruction of the appendix
  - (3) a softer stool may also help prevent diverticulitis
- c. helps prevent colon cancer
  - (1) the risk of colon cancer in countries in which people consume low-fat and high-fiber diets is 80–90 percent lower than the U.S. rate.
  - (2) fiber encourages production of mucus secreted from the intestinal wall, which forms a protective barrier against cancer-causing agents

     7.   the more a food is processed, the less fiber it usually contains

IX. Protein
- A. Composed of strings of amino acids
  1. twenty amino acids are needed by the body
     - a. eleven, called nonessential amino acids, can be produced by the body
     - b. nine, called essential amino acids, must be obtained through food
  2. foods that contain all nine essential proteins are called complete proteins
  3. foods that contain only some of the nine essential amino acids are called incomplete proteins
     - a. all essential amino acids must be present simultaneously for the body to make protein; careful pairing of incomplete proteins at the same meal will accomplish this (e.g., wheat bread and peanut butter)
- B. The human body is approximately 12–15 percent protein, most of it found in muscle
  1. structural proteins are found in muscle, hair, nails, tendons, ligaments
  2. globular proteins are found in almost 2000 enzymes
- C. How much protein should be consumed?
  1. protein should constitute 10–12 % of the diet
  2. some people erroneously think more is better
     - a. excessive protein is converted into fat, not muscle, with the excess nitrogen excreted in the urine which strains the kidneys

             b.   excess protein may also cause the body to excrete large amounts of calcium

             c.   there is some evidence that excess protein contributes to heart disease, osteoporosis, and accelerated growth of tumors.

             d.   people trying to build muscle mass need more carbohydrates, not more protein

    3.   To calculate the number of grams of protein you need each day, multiply your body weight in kilograms (pounds x 2.2) by 0.8 grams.

    4.   Pregnant women or women nursing infants are encouraged to increase protein consumption an extra 20 to 30 grams a day.

  D.   Protein is a source of energy for the body.

    1.   fat and carbohydrates are the primary sources of energy for the body, but some protein is used to produce energy

    2.   2–5 % of the body's resting energy comes from protein

    3.   as much as 10–15 % of the body's energy comes from protein during moderate and intense levels of physical activity

    4.   more protein will be broken down if insufficient carbohydrate is available

    5.   athletes who wish to maintain or build muscle mass need to consume the recommended amount of protein (10–12%) along with a high-carbohydrate diet

  E.   Vegetarian diets

    1.   types of vegetarians:

             a.   strict vegetarians or "vegans" do not eat any animal products including milk, meat, poultry or egg products

             b.   lactovegetarians exclude meat and eggs but consume dairy products

             c.   lacto-ovo-vegetarians exclude meat but include eggs and dairy products in their diet.

    2.   vegetarians, especially vegans, must carefully plan their diets to get all the essential amino acids through complementary incomplete protein foods

    3.   vegetarians have lower blood cholesterol, lower blood pressure, lower body fat, and reduced rates of coronary heart disease and lower mortality rates than nonvegetarians

    4.   the food pyramid has shifted a little closer to a vegetarian diet by emphasizing plant foods at the bottom two levels of the pyramid

X.   Vitamins

  A.   organic substances that are essential in small quantities

  B.   act in the regulation of body processes without providing energy or acting as building blocks

    1.   vitamins are part of enzymes and other substances which help regulate body processes

    2.   without vitamins, processes such as the production of hormones, antibodies, tissues, energy and blood coagulation would be impaired

  C.   vitamin deficiencies are rare in developed countries where a variety of foods is available

  D.   types of vitamins classified by the way they are processed in the body:

    1.   water-soluble

             a.   can dissolve in water

             b.   cannot be stored for extended periods of time, need to eat daily

             c.   excesses are excreted in urine

             d.   large doses generally do not pose a health threat as they are excreted

    2.   fat-soluble

             a.   A, D, E, K

        b.   do not dissolve in water, may be stored in body fat

        c.   daily consumption is not required since they can be stored

        d.   large doses of A and D can accumulate and become toxic

E.   RDA guidelines vary for age, gender, size, health status, activity level, and environment

    1.   a megadose is an excess of 10 times the RDA (recommended dietary allowance)

    2.   vitamins A and D should be limited to five and two times the RDA, respectively

F.   vitamin supplements

    1.   advertisers would have everyone believe that they need supplementation

    2.   most experts agree that if you are a healthy person eating a balanced diet, you do not need vitamin supplements

    3.   persons who need supplements include:

        a.   people with a medically determined need for a specific vitamin

        b.   pregnant and lactating women

        c.   people with erratic diets or unusual lifestyles like alcoholics or drug abusers

        d.   people in medically supervised low-calorie diets

        e.   elderly people who are not consuming a balanced diet

        f.   newborn infants (vitamin K to prevent excess bleeding)

G.   vitamins and disease prevention

    1.   research being done on vitamins and cancer, colds, heart disease and aging

    2.   research evidence of lower rates of cancer and heart disease among people who consumed greater than average quantities of vitamins C, E and A (beta carotene)

    3.   vitamins C, E, and A have the ability to reduce premature cell destruction caused by oxygen

        a.   oxygen that loses one too many electrons during the process of liberating energy from carbohydrates and fats is called a free radical

        b.   free radicals search for an electron and when they take one from another atom a new free radical is formed that goes looking for an electron—this chain of stealing electrons continues throughout the body, causing damage to lipids, proteins, cell walls, and even DNA

        c.   experts believe that free radicals may be responsible for premature aging, heart disease and cancer

        d.   the chain of electron stealing continues until one free radical meets another and combines or the free radical meets an antioxidant

        e.   vitamins C, E, and A are capable of acting as antioxidants

        f.   antioxidants can prevent the chain of electron stealing or slow it down long enough for two free radicals to meet

        g.   antioxidant research is based on consuming foods that contain vitamins C, A, and E, not supplements of these vitamins; not known if the food or just the vitamin plays the antioxidant role; supplements without other nutrients from the food may or may not be effective

XI.   Minerals

    A.   Inorganic compounds that facilitate chemical processes in the body, often becoming chemical structures of many of the products of the process

    B.   Require continual renewal

    C.   Important to:

      1.   the structure of teeth and bones

      2.   muscle contraction

      3.   neural activity

      4.   maintaining heart rhythm and acid-base balance in the body

      5.   enzymes and hormones, components of

      6.   the breaking down of fats, proteins, and carbohydrates

D.   Types:

      1.   macrominerals: more than 5 grams found in the body; known physiological function

      2.   trace minerals: need less than 100 mg a day

E.   Owing to abundance of minerals in food and small quantity needed, illnesses and diseases related to mineral deficiencies are rare

      1.   calcium, iron, and sodium may pose a threat to health

F.   Calcium

      1.   primary structural support for bone

      2.   RDA for adolescents and young adults is 1200 mg (four 8-ounce glasses of milk)

      3.   more than 75% of adults consume less than the daily requirement

      4.   about 25 % of women in the U.S. consume less than 300 mg of calcium a day

      5.   lack of calcium can result in osteoporosis (brittle, porous, weakened bones)

          a.   osteoporosis afflicts 24 million Americans and is responsible for one and a half million bone fractures annually

          b.   4 out of 5 people with osteoporosis are women; one out of five are men

          c.   can prevent through lifestyle habits early in life (birth to age 35)

               (1)   diet rich in calcium

               (2)   no smoking

               (3)   weight-bearing exercise

               (4)   moderate or no alcohol consumption

          d.   too much exercise can interfere with the menstrual cycle and estrogen production, which in turn can interfere with bone mass development

          e.   tobacco use and alcohol interfere with the absorption of calcium

          f.   vitamin D assists in the absorption of calcium

          g.   estrogen and hormone replacement therapy helps treat and prevent osteoporosis, especially helpful to postmenopausal women or women who have had their ovaries surgically removed

          h.   best plan: build strong bones early in life so that the slow depletion of them will not affect you later in life

G.   Iron

      1.   iron deficiency usually caused by failure to consume enough and by losses through regular menstrual bleeding

          a.   30–50 % of women fail to consume sufficient iron

      2.   vital role in oxygen-carrying capacity of blood and muscle

          a.   hemoglobin uses 80% of body's iron supply

      3.   low levels of iron over time deplete iron reserves and results in diminished oxygen-carrying capability

          a.   women may suffer from iron deficiency anemia

                (1)   general sluggishness

(2)   loss of appetite

(3)   susceptibility to infections

(4)   shortened attention span

(5)   impaired learning abilities

(6)   reduced capacity for even mild exercise

4.   RDA for iron is 10 and 15 milligrams for men and women respectively

5.   two sources:

      a.   plant: only 2–10 % of iron from plants is absorbed by the body

          (1)   red kidney beans, vegetables, Cream of Wheat good sources

      b.   animals: 10–35 % of iron from animal foods is absorbed

          (1)   lean beef products are good sources

6.   supplement only if diet doesn't provide adequate amounts; women tend to be deficient more than men

H.   Sodium

1.   recommended daily levels range from 1,100 to 3,000 milligrams

2.   salt contains 40 % sodium by weight; a teaspoon of salt= 2,000 mg

3.   disease relating to too much sodium in the diet

      a.   5 to 10 % of people are salt-sensitive meaning a high sodium diet can be responsible for elevated levels of blood pressure and related diseases including strokes and heart and kidney disease

      b.   difficult to determine who is salt sensitive so if all people consume a safe amount of salt the 5 to 10 % will be included

4.   sources:

      a.   processed foods: canned soup, cheese, chips, dried or smoked meats, prepared vegetables, pickles and even chocolate pudding

      b.   fast foods: large amounts added to many products

5.   guidelines for reducing sodium intake:

      a.   taste before salting foods

      b.   use alternate seasonings

      c.   eat natural vs. processed foods

      d.   avoid high sodium foods like smoked meats (bacon, sausage, ham)

      e.   reduce intake of canned and instant soups or eat low-sodium versions

      f.   read labels on all foods and select those with lower amounts of sodium

XII.   Water: the most vital nutrient

A.   All metabolic processes are conducted in an environment that contains water.

B.   Body is about 60% water by weight.

C.   Water has a variety of functions including:

1.   main ingredient of body fluids such as blood and lymph

2.   water-based synovial fluid surrounds joints and acts as a lubricant

3.   aids digestion of food and removal of waste products

4.   helps control body temperature

5.   involved in the sensation of balance and movement

D.   The body needs a constant supply of water.

E.   Sources of water:

1.   fluids we drink

          2.   foods we eat

              a.   fruit is 80 % water

              b.   bread, cheese, meats, vegetables, butter—lesser amounts

    F.   Water is lost through sweat, urine, feces, and evaporation in the lungs.

    G.   Need about 8 cups of fluids per day; varies with temperature and person's size and exertion.

    H.   Thirst indicates a need for fluids but may not represent the full need.

          1.   during exercise body needs larger than normal amounts of water

          2.   hot and humid climates increase the need for water intake

    I.   Heat stroke and heat exhaustion can occur with inadequate hydration.

XIII.   Current trends in eating

    A.   Fast food

          1.   one out of five Americans eats at a fast-food restaurant each day

          2.   food tends to be high in fat, sodium and protein and low in fiber and complex carbohydrates

          3.   taste and convenience sell the food, not necessarily good nutrition

          4.   careful selection of fast foods can result in a nutritious meal

          5.   restaurants will sell what the public wants—your selections determine the market

    B.   Snacking

          1.   snacking is not necessarily bad; smaller meals spread through the day can be good

          2.   problem is that most Americans choose high fat, high sodium foods to snack on

          3.   limit "taste good snacks" and include healthy snacks

XIV.   Food labels: truth and deception

    A.   FDA requires all food manufacturers to provide easy-to-understand nutritional information labels on products to which one or more additional nutrients have been added, or for which some nutritional claim has been made. Certain words are now also regulated by the FDA, words like "lean" and "light."

          1.   example of a food label (see overheads)

          2.   example of other food labels such as "light" and "lean" (see overhead)

    B.   Calculating fat using the food label (remember that fat contains 9 calories per gram).

          1.   a food containing 6 grams of fat contains 54 calories of fat (6 gm x 9 cal/gm)

          2.   a food with 6 gm of fat and a total of 100 calories contains 54 calories of fat; is 54% fat (54 calories divided by 100 calories = 0.54 or 54% fat)

XV.   Exercise and nutrition

    A.   Basic nutritional needs are the same for athletes and non-athletes; however, depending on the sport and the duration of the activity, some athletes may need to alter their diets to provide additional nutrients.

    B.   Energy for physical activity is supplied by the glucose in the blood stream and glycogen stored in the muscles and liver.

          1.   long-duration activity can deplete stores of glucose and glycogen

               a.   called "hitting the wall"

               b.   results in fatigue, decrease in performance, weakness, maybe dizziness, in extreme cases collapse

               c.   to prevent carbohydrate (glucose, glycogen) depletion, athletes do what is called carbohydrate loading

                    (1)   only recommended for persons involved in high-intensity endurance

activities that last a minimum of eighty continuous minutes
- (2) four days before event gradually reduce activity and consume a diet of 70% carbohydrates; body stores 2–3 times the normal amount of glucose
- (3) stored energy helps person maintain a level of intensity for longer

    C. Hydration is critical to athletic performance.
- 1. water is generally the best fluid during activity
- 2. sport drinks
  - a. no advantages for the person who needs fluid replacement
  - b. some advantages for long-term exercise
    - (1) added glucose used for energy during long hours of exercise
    - (2) minerals aid in water absorption
  - c. balanced diet gives average active persons all the glucose and minerals they need

XVI. Guidelines for healthy eating from a committee of experts brought together by the U.S. Department of Agriculture and the Department of Health and Human Services (1989).
- A. Eat a variety of foods.
- B. Maintain a healthy body weight.
- C. Consume a diet low in fat, saturated fat, and cholesterol.
- D. Eat plenty of vegetables, fruits, and grain products.
- E. Use sugars in moderation.
- F. Use salt and sodium in moderation.
- G. If you drink alcohol, do so in moderation (moderation is 2 drinks a day for men, 1 drink a day for women).

XVII. Making long-term dietary changes
- A. Assessment
  - 1. Before you can make a change, you need to assess your diet and determine which nutrients you are getting enough of, too little of, and too much of.
  - 2. Use Lab 6.2 for a three-day diet analysis.
- B. A plan of action
  - 1. select one small area of change
  - 2. make change gradually, allowing for taste and habit adjustment
  - 3. plan ahead which foods you will eat
  - 4. dine out wisely
    - a. ask for sauces and dressings on the side
    - b. avoid fried foods and fatty meats
    - c. limit the number of times you eat out
  - 5. analyze your favorite dishes
    - a. if high in fat, etc., try to reduce the number or size of servings
    - b. look for low-fat alternatives such as frozen yogurt in place of ice cream

BEHAVIOR BOOSTS: STAGE-BASED STUDENT ACTIVITIES

Precontemplator

- Take strength in knowing that you're not alone. In one survey 31 percent of individuals were precontemplators when it comes to eating a low-fat diet.
- Name one good reason for changing the way you eat.
- Ask several people who have changed their diets why they did it and how they're feeling.
- Think about the reasons you eat what you eat.
- Young adults carry eating habits into adulthood. Think about the effect a lifetime of poor eating could have on your health.

Contemplator
- The next time you are at a fast-food restaurant, pick up a brochure that lists the nutritional content of their menu selections.
- Find out which fruits and vegetables are currently in season. These will be the best-tasting fruits and vegetables.
- When you are tempted to eat high-fat foods, think of all the reasons not to.

Preparer
- Compare the food label of a low-fat food version of a food you regularly eat (such as mayonnaise) to that of a normal product. Calculate the amount of fat you will eliminate in your diet if you use the low-fat version during the following week.
- Buy a healthy diet cookbook and try one new recipe every week.
- Changing your diet is hard. Today, try changing just your lunch.
- Read the labels on everything you eat in one day.

Action Taker
- In restaurants and cafeterias, select items with the "healthy heart" logo.
- Substitute one low-fat product for the regular food (skim milk for regular milk, low-fat mayonnaise or salad dressing for regular.)
- Steam or stir-fry your vegetables rather than boiling them or serving them with sauces.
- Plan and prepare a week's menu of healthy meals.
- If you buy meat, select lean cuts.

Maintainer
- Devise a plan for continuing healthy eating during busy weeks and while traveling.
- Share your lunch with a precontemplator.
- Try new fruits and vegetables and low-fat alternatives to keep your diet varied and interesting.

RESOURCES

Suggested Reading

Beasley, J.D., and J. Swift. 1989. *The Kellogg Report: The Impact on Nutrition, Environment & Lifestyle on the Health of Americans.* Annadale-on-Hudson, NY: Institute of Health Policy and Practice, the Bard College Center.

74

Clark, N. 1991. Now to pack a meatless diet full of nutrients. *The Physician and Sports Medicine.* 19:31.

Cutler, R.G., 1991. Antioxidants and aging. *American Journal of Clinical Nutrition* 53:3735.

Filer, L.J. 1991. Recommended dietary allowances: How did we get where we are? *Nutrition Today,* September/October.

Geiger, C.J. 1991. Review of nutrition labeling formats. *Journal of American Dietetic Association* 91(7):805-11.

Hertzler, A.A., and R.B. Fray. 1989. Food behavior of college students. *Adolescence.* 24(94):349-350.

Organizations

American Institute of Nutrition
9650 Rockville Pike
Bethesda, MD 20814

Center for Science in the Public Interest
1875 Connecticut Avenue, NW, Suite 300
Washington, D.C. 20009

Community Systems Foundation
1130 Hill Street
Ann Arbor, MI 48104

Food and Nutrition Information Center
National Agricultural Library
10301 Baltimore Blvd.
Beltsville, MD 20705

Human Nutrition Information Service
United States Department of Agriculture
Hyattsville, MD 20782

Films and Videos

A Practical Approach to a High-Fiber Diet. This film defines dietary fiber and discusses the relationship between various diseases and fiber intake. Videotape.

Carbo Choices: A Quiz on Carbohydrates. The program's quiz format provides and answers to typical consumer questions about carbohydrates—fiber, starch, and sugar. Helps viewers make the healthy dietary choices. Videotape.

Audio-Visual Services
Pennsylvania State University
Special Services Building
1127 Fox Hill Road
University Park, PA 16803-1824
(800) 826-0132

Cholesterol: What You Can Do. Discusses the various foods we need to be concerned about.

Alfred Higgins Productions
6530 Laurel Canyon Road
Hollywood, CA 91606

Weighing the Choices: Positive Approaches to Nutrition. Program presents practical nutritious dietary alternatives, not to totally replace certain foods in the diet but to give the individual the opportunity to improve diet with little difficulty or disruption. Videotape.

The Altschul Group
930 Pitner Avenue
Evanston, IL 60202
(800) 421-2363

Additional Local and Community Resources

American Heart Association
Blue Cross/Blue Shield (booklet: *Food and Fitness: Blueprint for Health*, vol 24; charge.)
Dairy Council, state and local (leaflet: *Guide to Good Eating*)
Dietetic Association (state)

Understanding Body Composition

Chapter 7

CHAPTER SUMMARY

A major threat to good health and wellness is excessive body fat. Though it is necessary to have some fat, too much can contribute to the risk of heart disease, diabetes, and cancer. All the components of the human body can be classified as either lean body weight or fat. The amount and location of body fat can be measured using height and weight charts or by indirect estimation of total body fat using skin calipers, hydrostatic weighing, or bioelectric impedance, among other methods. Once the amount of body fat is known, it is possible to calculate ideal body weight. Individuals who have body weights at, or near, ideal tend to be somewhat protected from the disease associated with excessive body fat.

LEARNING OBJECTIVES

The student will be able to:
- define lean body weight and fat weight.
- explain the functions of fat in the body.
- distinguish between essential and nonessential body fat.
- differentiate between subcutaneous, intramuscular and cellulite fat.
- identify gender differences concerning amounts of fat and locations of stored fat.
- identify the health risks associated with different body shapes.
- describe the five health classifications for body fat.
- describe the dangers of obesity.
- assess risk of obesity using body mass index (BMI).
- describe three methods of measuring body fat.
- calculate ideal body weight.
- measure and evaluate body shape and body fat.
- explain the roles of exercise and diet in lowering percentage of body fat.

PERSONAL PROFILE

See the profiles for chapters 6 (Striving for Wellness with Proper Nutrition) and 8 (Controlling Body Weight).

CONTENT OUTLINE

I. Health risk is related to body shape and body composition
    A. Body length and shape is determined primarily by the genes you inherit.
        1. people with large, heavier upper bodies have greater health risk than people who have thin upper bodies
        2. there are several methods for determining health risk based on body shape
    B. Body composition has to do with the percentages of fat and lean body weight you possess.
        1. all tissues can be categorized as either fat or lean body weight
            a. fat weight (FW) is that percentage of your total body that is fat.
            b. lean body mass (LBM) is the portion of your body weight that is not fat, such as the muscles, skin, hair, bone, blood, other organs, all other nonfat tissues.
        2. too much fat weight increases health risk
        3. amount of fat weight is largely determined by:
            a. heredity
            b. diet
            c. physical activity

II. Types of body fat
    A. Essential body fat
        1. the minimum percent of body fat needed for normal physiological function
            a. approximately 5 % for men, 8% for women
        2. provides energy and building materials
        3. surrounds organs and acts as padding
    B. Nonessential fat
        1. any fat in excess of that required for normal physiological function
        2. excessive amounts are unhealthy
    C. Subcutaneous fat
        1. fat stored just under the skin
        2. more stored in some areas than others (eg., abdomen vs. back of hand)
    D. Intramuscular fat
        1. fat stored in the muscle
        2. supplies energy to muscles for sustained physical activity
    E. Cellulite
        1. fat under the skin where the skin isn't as tight
        2. fat is trapped in the connective tissues that attach your skin to the underlying muscle
        3. dimpled areas are where the skin is more firmly attached to the muscle
        4. differences in skin thickness and arrangement of connective tissue make cellulite appear in more women than men
        5. some cellulite cannot be removed even with proper diet and exercise

III. Gender differences
    A. Women need more fat for childbearing purposes.
    B. Women tend to store fat in the hips, thighs, and breasts.
    C. Men tend to store fat in the abdomen, chest and back.
    D. Women with too little fat may develop amenorrhea (menstruation ceases).
        1. happens to some athletes including dancers, and women with eating disorders

    2.   too little fat affects estrogen production and lowers calcium absorption

    3.   may cause bone density loss which can lead to osteoporosis later in life

    4.   when essential fat weight is restored, menstruation, estrogen production and calcium absorption resume

IV.   Functions of body fat

    A.   Storage of energy

        1.   each gram of fat has 9 calories that can be used for muscle contraction or other metabolic functions

        2.   without stored fat we would have to eat constantly to sustain proper body functioning

        3.   enables survival during prolonged periods of starvation

    B.   Padding

        1.   protection against injury and trauma

        2.   provides shock absorption

    C.   Insulation

        1.   fat contains less water than muscle; therefore, it is a better form of insulation

        2.   helps maintain body temperature

V.   Percent body fat is the amount of your total weight that is fat weight.

    A.   Persons of different weights can have the same percentage body fat.

    B.   The percentage of body fat a person has is a good indicator of health risk.

    C.   Percentage body fat is a better indicator of risk than body weight.

VI.   Obesity

    A.   More than 25 percent fat for men and 32 percent fat for women

    B.   More than 20 percent above the ideal body weight as determined by a height and weight chart

VII. Overweight

    A.   More than 10 percent above the ideal body weight as determined by a weight and height chart

    B.   Measures of overweightness are rough estimates of body composition and should not be used to determine weight-loss goals.

    C.   Muscular individuals can be "overweight" but actually have a good percentage of body fat.

    D.   Some individuals with near ideal weights can have high percentages of body fat.

VIII. Body fat distribution

    A.   Android, or apple, body shape has more fat around the abdominal area than hips or thighs.

        1.   more common among men than women

        2.   associated with a higher risk of disease

    B.   Gynoid, or pear, body type has fat deposits mostly on the hips and thighs.

        1.   more common among women than men

        2.   pear body type has a slender upper body and small breasts

        3.   after menopause (decrease in estrogen) fat tends to be stored in the typical android locations

    C.   Neutral body shape

    D.   Most people are a combination of android and gynoid body shapes.

    E.   The android body type has a higher prevalence of heart disease, stroke, cancer and diabetes. Possible reasons include:

        1.   abdominal fat cells are larger than other fat cells and they have an intolerance for blood sugars and insulin which increases the likelihood of diabetes developing

        2.   excessive insulin interferes with kidney function, which leads to high blood pressure, which is a risk factor for a number of cardiovascular diseases

3. abdominal fat cells have high levels of fat-mobilizing enzymes that facilitate the removal and storage of fat

    a. rapid release and storage of fat from android locations cause blood cholesterol to rise which in turn increases cardiovascular disease risk

    b. android fat is easy to put on and take off; gynoid fat is much more difficult to take off

F. To measure body shape and determine risk of heart disease take a ratio of the circumference of the waist and hip and refer to Lab 7.1 on page 189.

IX. Health classifications for body fat

A. Excessively lean: < 8 % women, < 5 % men

1. unhealthy, may be due to illness, eating disorder, a very low-calorie restricted diet, or prolonged endurance-type activities on a regular basis

2. associated with insufficient intake of energy and muscle wasting (protein pulled from muscle to use for energy)

3. other symptoms: fatigue, amenorrhea, and loss of bone mass

4. society places a strong emphasis on outward appearance, sometimes leading to unhealthy habits as people try to reach unrealistic "fashionable body types"

B. Lean: 8–17 % women, 5–9 % men

1. associated with people involved in high performance athletics

2. healthy as long as a proper diet is maintained

C. Healthy: 18–25 % women, 10–20% men

1. recommended level of fat for most adults

2. health risks associated with too much and too little body fat are minimized

D. Moderately Overfat: 26–32 % women, 21–25 % men

1. gradually increasing risk for cancer, heart disease, and diabetes

E. Obese: > 32 % women, > 25 % men

1. the higher the degree of overfatness, the higher the risk of disease and premature death

    a. high blood pressure is 3 times more common among the obese, including school aged children

    b. may have elevated levels of blood cholesterol and blood fats

    c. significantly higher rates of heart disease

    d. diabetes is 3 times more common

    e. men have higher rates of colon, rectal and prostate cancer

    f. women have higher rates of gallbladder, breast, cervical, uterine, and ovarian cancer

    g. premature death rate is 1–2 times higher than for average-weight people

2. psychological impact of obesity in a society that associates beauty, intelligence, and success with thinness

    a. social pressures may result in feelings of guilt, depression, low self-esteem, and anxiety

    b. adolescents are particularly vulnerable as self-esteem is developing and peers (who also lack self-esteem) can be cruel

    c. may also lead to psychological stress, reduced income, and discrimination both on the job and in personal life

80

X. Assessing risk of obesity
- A. Body Mass Index (BMI)
    1. see activity 7.1 on page 185
    2. body weight (in kilograms) divided by height squared
    3. based on concept that weight should be proportional to height
    4. more accurate than height/weight tables but does not distinguish fat from LBM
    5. fairly accurate for people without a lot of muscle mass
    6. ACSM states ideal BMI is 21–23 for women, 22–24 for men
    7. BMI greater than 27.8 for men, or 27.3 for women is associated with increased cardiovascular disease risk
    8. high BMIs are associated with hypertension, high blood cholesterol and triglycerides, and low levels of HDL
- B. Assessing body fat
    1. hydrostatic weighing (underwater weighing)
        a. one of the more accurate indirect measures of body fat
        b. person sits on a platform which is lowered into a tank of water to determine an underwater weight, adjustments are made for air trapped inside the body
        c. since fat floats, a lean person will weigh more underwater than a fat person
        d. fairly costly both in time and equipment
        e. only works well for those who are comfortable exhaling underwater
    2. skinfold method
        a. fairly accurate technique, less accurate than hydrostatic weighing
        b. estimates total body fat based on subcutaneous fat at various sites
        c. a skin caliper is used to measure the subcutaneous fat and then a formula used to estimate an overall percentage of body fat
        d. common sites are: back of the arm, above the hip, abdomen, below the shoulder blade, front of the thigh
        e. easy to perform, usually no cost or a nominal fee
    3. bioelectric impedance
        a. if hydration is held constant this method provides a fairly accurate estimate (similar to that of the skinfold technique)
        b. an impedance machine sends a small electrical charge through the body and records the amount of resistance or impedance the charge meets as it travels
        c. based on the idea that electricity hits more resistance going through fat than muscle (which is mostly water)
        d. because the test can be influenced by total body water, repeat tests must be given with the person at the same hydration levels (menstruation and exercise can affect hydration)
        e. electrodes are placed on the ankle and wrist, person doesn't feel anything
        f. computer printout provides a percentage of fat and also a recommended exercise/diet program

XI. Ideal body weight
- A. It should fall within a lean to healthy range of body fat.
- B. Where you choose to be along the range determines activity level, etc.
    1. a woman who wants to be 17% fat will need to perform regular vigorous exercise and eat a diet that is well balanced and can sustain this level of activity

2. a woman who is content with 25% fat will minimize health risks and be able to sustain this percentage of fat with less strenuous exercise and a less restrictive balanced diet

C. Calculations of ideal body weight:
  1. using height
    a. use when a measure of body fat is unavailable
    b. multiply height in inches by 3.5 (women) or 4.0 (men) and subtract 108 (women) or 128 (men).
    c. if you are large boned add 10% to the final figure
      (1) considered large boned if the wrist measurement on your dominant wrist exceeds 6.5 inches (women) or 7.0 inches (men)
  2. using percent body fat
    a. more accurate than estimate from height
    b. see Activity 7.2 to help calculate ideal body weight:
      (1) multiply your current body weight by your current % body fat to find out the number of pounds of fat you currently have
      (2) subtract the number of pounds from your current weight to find the number of lean body pounds you have
      (3) subtract your desired % body fat (ex. 0.19 for 19%) from 1.0
      (4) divide your lean body pounds by your answer from step 3 to determine your ideal weight in pounds

XII. Changing your percentage of body fat
  A. FW can be reduced through exercise and diet.
  B. LBM can be increased through resistance exercise.
  C. To determine the amount of change carefully consider lifestyle, health status, cultural and social values and personal desires.

BEHAVIOR BOOSTS: STAGED-BASED STUDENT ACTIVITIES

See the Behavior Boosts for chapter six (Striving for Wellness with Proper Nutrition) and chapter eight (Controlling Body Weight).

ADDITIONAL SUGGESTED STUDENT ACTIVITIES

Activity 1: Body Mass Index (BMI)
Determine health risk by calculating BMI using the directions in Activity 7.1 on page 185 in the text.

Activity 2: Ideal Body Weight
Calculate ideal body weight from height using the directions on page 186 in the text.
Calculate ideal body weight from weight and percent body fat using Activity 7.2 on page 187 of the text.

Activity 3: Field Trip

Travel to a facility that performs body fat measurements. This facility may be an on-campus exercise science lab or an off-campus facility.

LABS

Lab 7.1 What is Your Body Shape? See the photographs on page 182 and the lab on page 189.
Lab 7.2 Measuring Body Fat Using the Skinfold Method, pages 190-192

RESOURCES

Suggested Reading

American College of Sports Medicine (L. Durstine, et.al. eds*.), Resource Manual for Guidelines for Exercise Testing and Prescription*, Second Edition. Lea and Febiger, Philadelphia, 1993.

American Council on Exercise. *Personal Trainer Manual*: The Resource for Fitness Instructors. San Diego, CA: American Council on Exercise, 1991.

Bruch, H. *Eating disorders*. New York: Basic Books, 1973.

Katch, F.I., and W.D. McArdle. *Nutrition, weight control, and exercise*, 3rd ed. Philadelphia: Lea & Febiger, 1988.

Organizations

American Alliance of Health, Physical Education, Recreation and Dance (AAHPERD)
1900 Association Drive
Reston, VA 20191-1599
Tel (800) 213-7193
E-mail: info@aahperd.org
Web site: http://www.aahperd.org

American College of Sports Medicine (ACSM)
P.O. Box 1440
Indianapolis, IN 46206-1440
Tel (317) 637-9200
Fax (317) 634-7817
Web site: http://www.acsm.org
American Council on Exercise (ACE)
6190 Cornerstone Court, East, Suite 202
San Diego, CA 92121-4729
5820 Oberlin Drive. Suite 102
San Diego. CA 92121-3787

Tel (619) 535-8227
Fax (619) 535-1778
Web site: http://www.ACEfitness.org

American Medical Athletic Association (AMAA)
4405 East West Highway
Suite 405
Bethesda, MD 20804
Tel: (800) 776-2732
Web site: http://www.arfa.org/amaa

President's Council on Physical Fitness and Sports (PCPFS)
450 Fifth Street, NW, Suite 7103
Washington. DC 20001
(202) 272-2451
Web site: http://www.hhs.gov/progorg/ophs/pcpfs

Video

Fitness for Life: Body Composition. Looks at the relationship between exercise and body composition through discussion of weight control via diet and exercise. 29 minutes, videotape.

Additional Local and Community Resources

American Heart Association
Blue Cross/Blue Shield
County Recreation Departments
Governor's Council on Health and Fitness
Jewish Community Center
State and County Health Departments
YMCA and YWCA

Audio-Visual Services
Pennsylvania State University, Special Services
Building
1127 Fox Hill Road
University Park, PA 16803-1824
(800) 826-0132

Controlling Body Weight

Chapter 8

CHAPTER SUMMARY

Despite increases in physical activity and an improved overall diet, Americans are more overweight now than ever before. Obesity directly contributes to several disease and other health conditions. It is caused by a combination of three interrelated factors: cultural influences, genetics, and lifestyle, and no one theory can explain why individuals gain and lose weight. Increased social and emotional pressures can force some individuals to become victims of equally dangerous eating disorders. Successful weight loss and maintenance requires a lifelong commitment to healthy eating and regular physical activity.

LEARNING OBJECTIVES

The student will be able to:
- describe the prevalence and seriousness of being overweight or obese.
- explain how excessive body fat can affect health.
- explain the energy balance and set point theories of weight gain.
- explain how genetics, metabolism, and adiposity can contribute to obesity.
- describe and identify eating disorders.
- outline an appropriate weight-loss and weight-maintenance strategy.
- distinguish a healthy weight-loss program from a fad or get-rich-quick program.
- explain why a program of diet and exercise is the best method to lose weight and maintain weight loss.

PERSONAL PROFILE

Oprah the "Maintainer"

In 1991, the word was out. After a sensational weight loss victory, Oprah Winfrey was on national TV promoting the use of Slim Fast as a fantastic way to lose weight. After all, it helped her lose an amazing seventy pounds and she looked great. However, within months the media was quick to report that the celebrity was once again back at her original weight of 222 pounds and then some. Oprah had given all of America a graphic example of yo-yo dieting, defined as rapid weight loss followed by rapid weight gain.

Oprah has never been one to give up easily. For the next several years she struggled using different dieting techniques to try to reduce her body weight. Finally, in March 1993, she called Bob Greene, a personal trainer, and asked him to help. The goal this time was to use healthy weight-loss methods to lose 72 pounds and maintain her body weight at a reasonable 150 pounds. That meant regular aerobic exercise combined with changes in diet to produce gradual weight loss. This time the changes in Oprah's lifestyle would need to be permanent and she was determined to do it.

Each day at 5 A.M., the workouts began. At first, Oprah's workouts consisted of a 2½ mile walk, soon mixed with a little jogging. Within two weeks, she was running or walking for three or four miles. In the afternoons, she would also climb onto her Stairmaster for forty-five minutes and lift weights for thirty minutes. "That is probably too aggressive a program for most people," Greene admits, "but I wanted to get her metabolism revved up." Days turned into weeks and weeks into months as Oprah started losing between eight and ten pounds a month. It didn't take long for her to reach her desired weight. Her exercise schedule was reduced to one run a day and Oprah set her sights on her next goal, the Marine Corps Marathon.

After averaging around fifty miles per week for three months, she ran the first marathon of her life. She covered the 26-mile distance without walking a single step. Some have said that Oprah has it easy because she has her own personal trainer and chef. "That's not true," says Greene. "When she's getting ready to run at 5 A.M. or she is out there pounding the pavement, no one can run for her." The changes Oprah has made in her life are due to her determination to succeed and not because of someone else's prodding. Bob Green would like to think that her progress and her commitment will show millions of other people that they, too, can improve their lives.

Adapted from Lamb, L. The Oprah Winfrey syndrome, *Health Letter* 37(7):1-2, 1991, and Reynolds, G. The Oprah Winfrey plan. *Runner's World*, 64-66, March 1995.

CONTENT OUTLINE

I.   Americans are the most overfat people in the world, with one-quarter of the population considered to be clinically obese.

II.   Over half of men (56%) and three quarters of women (78%) are unhappy with their current weight.
    A.   33 billion dollars are spent on weight-loss
       1.   few lasting results
       2.   money is spent on thigh creams, liquid drinks, diet pills, fashion diets, and commercial diet programs
    B.   At any given time 24% of men and 40% of women are engaged in some type of weight-loss method

III. The desire to be "thin" is fueled more by vanity and social acceptance than health.
    A.   Fewer than one-half of the women who diet actually need to lose weight.
    B.   Only one out of ten women diets because of health reasons.
    C.   Unrealistic expectations about body weight and shape can result in eating disorders, diet anxiety, and added health risk.

IV.   Theories concerning weight gain
    A.   The energy balance theory of weight gain suggests that extra fat is stored when more energy is consumed than is expended.
       1.   infants have high energy intake and low energy output (mostly sedentary) and therefore have more body fat than any other group; as activity increases their body fat decreases

        2.   between the ages of 20 and 60 men typically increase from 15 to 25% fat, women from 20 to 32%

            a.   may be called "age onset obesity"

            b.   changes in diet, exercise (activity level), metabolism and body composition can all contribute to the increase in body fat with age

    B.   The set point theory holds that the body has a preference for a certain weight (its "set point") and defends that weight against weight loss or weight gain. Proponents believe:

        1.   the set point is partly determined by genetics

        2.   the only effective way to lower the set point is through daily physical activity

    C.   Neither theory fully explains why fat is gained but evidence suggests the need for calorie restrictions and regular physical activity.

V.   Energy expenditure is determined by two main factors: metabolism and physical activity.

VI.   Metabolism is the sum of all vital body processes by which food, energy, and nutrients are made available to, and used by, the body.

    A.   Total metabolism = the resting metabolic rate (RMR) + the energy required to digest and use food and perform physical movement.

        1.   RMR represents the energy required to maintain vital functions at rest.

        2.   RMR represents about 55–75% of all expended energy (about 1,650 calories)

            a.   see Activity 8.1 to calculate your resting metabolic rate

        3.   energy to digest food represents about 5–15% of all expended energy

            a.   complex carbohydrates and protein require more energy to metabolize than simple sugars

            b.   the caloric content of one gram of protein is 5.6 but 1.6 calories are used to metabolize it which leaves 4 calories available

    B.   Metabolic rate is influenced by genetics, age, illness, stimulants and exercise.

        1.   high metabolic rates can be inherited or the result of a hyperactive thyroid

        2.   women typically have lower metabolic rates than men

        3.   muscle increases metabolic rate; every pound of muscle requires 30–60 calories per day just for maintenance

        4.   metabolic rate decreases with age but this is probably related to losses in muscle mass

        5.   rapid weight gains and losses can result in a more efficient metabolic system

            a.   body conserves calories by becoming more efficient

            b.   takes fewer calories to maintain body functions

            c.   weight becomes harder to lose and easier to gain

        6.   stimulants such as nicotine and caffeine increase resting metabolic rate temporarily

            a.   caffeine is often an ingredient of diet pills and drinks

            b.   some people smoke to decrease their appetites so they can lose weight

VII. Factors that are responsible for individual differences in body fat.

    A.   Genetic factors are responsible for about 25% of the variation among individuals.

        1.   people inherit their metabolism, number of fat cells, etc.

        2.   children of obese children are more apt to be obese; could be genetics or lifestyle

        3.   adopted children tend to have body weights and shapes similar to their biological parents rather than their adoptive parents

    B.   Cultural factors are responsible for about 30% of the variation among individuals.

        1.   choice of foods including holiday foods

        2.   people tend to eat what their parents cook and eat

  C.   Other factors like lifestyle and environment are responsible for about 45% of the variation among individuals.

VIII.   Factors that influence obesity

  A.   Genetics usually plays only a small role in the overall cause of obesity.

        1.   recent research suggests that a genetic disorder may be partially responsible for added weight gain in some people

        2.   this genetic disorder is rare

  B.   The environmental, cultural and lifestyle factors that influence what and how we eat and whether or not we participate in regular physical activity are the greatest causes of obesity.

        1.   advertisers and marketing campaigns sell lifestyles and foods that are conducive to obesity

        2.   high-tech world minimizes physical activity

IX.   Less than obese conditions of overfatness are also associated with disease.

        1.   individuals should use readings of percent body fat to determine a healthy body weight

        2.   only those individuals who are overfat should consider weight-loss

X.   Eating disorders

  A.   Anorexia nervosa

        1.   estimated that 1–3 million Americans suffer from this

           a.   mostly women

           b.   men can also be anorexic but the number of cases is small

        2.   associated with life-threatening weight losses and denial of weight loss by the dieter

           a.   self-starvation and exercise are used

           b.   causes malnutrition and nutrient deficiencies

           c.   as body fat becomes very low, internal organs normally supported by fat begin to sag and can gradually stop functioning

           d.   15–20% of anorexics die

        3.   American Psychiatric Association list of criteria for identifying those with anorexia (see text page 198)

        4.   causes for anorexia are complex

           a.   genetic factor—some evidence of anorexia among sets of sisters

           b.   women raised by domineering mothers

           c.   women who feel extreme cultural pressure to be thin

           d.   psychological nature of the disease makes it hard to find any one cause

        5.   treatment involves hospitalization, medications to stimulate appetite, and psychological counseling

           a.   anorexic individuals deny they have a problem

           b.   difficult to get into treatment

  B.   Bulimia

        1.   characterized by eating regular or large meals and then intentionally emptying the food out of the stomach by self-induced vomiting or use of laxatives

           a.   constant concern with body weight

           b.   regular secret eating (binges)

        c.   loss of control over eating habits during binging

        d.   at least 2 binges a week for at least 3 months

        e.   frequent purging

    2.   2–8 percent of adolescent and college-age women suffer from bulimia; affects men but is rare

    3.   dangers involved include: damage to the throat and esophagus from regurgitated stomach acids, erosion of tooth enamel, electrolyte imbalances, psychological problems including depression and anxiety

    4.   treatment: medical and psychological

XI.   Safe and successful weight-loss strategies are achieved through a combination of a balanced diet and exercise.

    A.   Exercise (see also chapters 2 and 3)

        1.   exercise aids weight loss by burning calories

        2.   aerobic exercise emphasizes fat loss

            a.   after 20 minutes of aerobic exercise 50% of the fuel for activity is fat

            b.   anaerobic exercise uses primarily carbohydrate for fuel

        3.   an intensity that can be maintained for 20–60 minutes

        4.   performed 6–7 days a week

        5.   formal exercise or informal physical activities like taking the stairs

        6.   to be successful must become a natural (habitual) part of a person's daily life

        7.   boosts resting metabolism so that more calories are burned after exercise

            a.   increase and/or maintenance of muscle mass requires calories which helps prevent the decrease in metabolism experienced with aging

            b.   increase in resting metabolism following exercise

                 (1)   not sure for how long the increase lasts but it expends about 15 calories per every 100 calories expended in physical activity

        8.   diet restrictions alone (no exercise) will decrease both body fat and muscle

        9.   diet and exercise combined result in weight loss from reduced body fat

    B.   Proper diet

        1.   to lose weight, more calories must be expended than taken in

        2.   total daily caloric intake should be reduced no more than 500 calories a day or 1,000 calories a day if your present diet exceeds 3,000 calories

        3.   consume a minimum of 1,200 calories

        4.   diet tips

            a.   eat planned meals

            b.   eat fiber-rich food

            c.   eat fresh fruits and vegetables

            d.   eat low-fat meats

            e.   limit number of times you eat out

            f.   write down what you eat

            g.   allow an occasional treat to avoid binges

            h.   make gradual changes in one or two areas

        5.   cutting fat

            a.   for weight loss can drop to 20% of diet vs. 30%

            b.   dietary fat has more influence than carbohydrates and proteins on body fat

   (1) takes less energy to digest fat than carbohydrates

   (2) fat is more easily stored

   (3) emphasize fruits and vegetables; de-emphasize meats, processed foods, fast foods, fried food, and some dairy products

   (4) read food labels for fat content

C. Very low calorie diets (VLCDs)

  1. prescribed for some obese people with body mass indexes greater than 30 kg/m^2

  2. limit total caloric intake to 400–800 calories a day

  3. medical supervision required, person often hospitalized or checked into a care facility

  4. used only when traditional weight loss methods have not worked

  5. success rate for losing the weight and maintaining an ideal weight is relatively low

D. Yo-yo or weight cycling diets

  1. characterized by repetitive losing and gaining of weight

  2. research is mixed as to whether this results in added health risk

E. The American College of Sports Medicine recommends a weight loss program that:

  1. has a diet consisting of no less than 1,200 calories

  2. includes foods acceptable to the dieter

  3. provides a negative calorie balance

  4. includes behavior modification techniques

  5. includes exercise

  6. provides that new eating and exercise habits be continued for life

F. The recommended safe weight loss is ½ to 1 pound per week.

  1. during the first 3 days 70% of weight loss is water, 25% is fat

   a. every stored gram of carbohydrate requires 3 grams of water be stored with it

   b. as carbohydrate stores are used up, the stored water is released

  2. plateaus may occur; continue with diet and exercise and weight loss will resume

G. Unbalanced diets

  1. those that stress one kind of food do not supply all the necessary nutrients

  2. high-protein diets do not provide the body with sufficient carbohydrate and fat for energy

   a. the metabolism of protein for energy has a by-product of nitrogen; high levels of nitrogen can be toxic

   b. in the kidneys nitrogen is joined with water to make ammonia and excreted; this requires a lot of water and few people drink sufficient water; may lead to dehydration and kidney failure

  3. high-protein diets often encourage meat and dairy products rich in saturated fats

  4. "all you can eat diets" often fail to encourage a balanced diet, and any type of food which brings in more calories than are expended will result in weight gain

H. Weight-loss myths

  1. promise quick, easy weight loss

  2. sound too good to be true

  3. require a substance with a secret ingredient

  4. limit you to a certain brand of food or products

  5. don't use a balanced diet or mix foods for a special effect

  6. claim that you can eat all you want

  7. don't encourage exercise

8. promise a 5 pound weight loss in the first week but fail to say it is a water loss
9. use plastic wrappings, rubber suits, and saunas to sweat off water weight
10. use waist and thigh belts to push water aside in order to take quick measurements that indicate a loss, pretending it is a fat loss
11. use vibrating machines, toning tables, and thigh creams to melt away fat
12. use mouth sprays or diet pills to decrease appetite

XII. Weight gain
   A. Is desired by individuals who are underweight due to illness or malnutrition, by individuals wishing to gain more mass (generally muscle mass), and by pregnant women.
   B. Requires an increase in caloric intake that exceeds caloric expenditure
      1. pregnant women should increase consumption about 300 calories a day
      2. for serious lean body mass gains, some experts recommend an increase of 700–1000 calories coupled with rigorous resistance
   C. Diet should maintain the recommended balance of fat, protein, and carbohydrate
      1. a common error is to increase the percentage of protein consumed resulting in insufficient carbohydrate and fat fuel for exercise and daily activity

XIII. Weight maintenance
   A. Studies of the long-term success rate of most diets concludes that only 5 % of dieters reach and maintain their target weight for more than one year.
   B. Requires a commitment to lifetime habits of proper eating and exercise.
   C. Requires that you adjust your diet as life demands change (change in activity, pregnancy, etc.).
   D. Tips to help maintain weight
      1. find exercise/physical activity you enjoy
      2. instead of buying bigger clothes, concentrate on keeping off the weight
      3. identify and minimize hunger triggers such as time of day, smell of food, stress, boredom, grocery shopping and advertisements
      4. surround yourself with social support (ask people to help you)
      5. expect to relapse and be prepared with a plan to begin again

BEHAVIOR BOOSTS: STAGE-BASED STUDENT ACTIVITIES

Precontemplator
- Put a picture of a person with a healthy looking body on your refrigerator.
- Take comfort in knowing precontemplators for weight loss usually move quickly to the contemplation stage.
- If you have previously tried to lose weight and failed, you are not alone. It is a difficult change to make. Sixty percent of adults are currently trying to control body fat.
- Think about the advantages of having a body with a healthy level of fat.

Contemplator
- Review the risks associated with excessive body fat.
- Review your nutrition analysis from Chapter 6 to see how many calories you consume each day.
- Discuss your weight-loss goals with someone who can support your efforts to lose weight.

- Talk to a few people who have maintained their weight loss. Ask them how they overcame their barriers.

Preparer
- Find a form of regular exercise that works for you. You don't have to be a marathon runner!
- Be patient when you first start an exercise program. Realize that it takes a while to see results.
- Let your friends and family know you want to lose weight and ask them to support you.
- Enroll in an exercise class and make it as important a part of your schedule as anything else you do.

Action Taker
- Commitment is everything. Commit yourself to changing your current lifestyle.
- Once you have lost some weight, keeping the weight off becomes your next goal. To help maintain your weight loss, jot down some ideas for a good diet.
- Think about the clothes that fit you better and how much better you look in them since you started controlling your body fat.
- Think of a new way to regard yourself for your hard work in taking action to control your weight.

Maintainer
- Make a plan for adjusting to the major changes in your life that could lead you to gain weight (for example, marriage, or a new job).
- Think of a new activity you would like to try if you get bored with your current activities.

ADDITIONAL STUDENT ACTIVITIES

Activity 1: Monitoring fat loss and body shape using body measurements.

It is possible to lose several pounds of body fat and still not lose total body weight. Exercise strengthens and often enlarges muscles. The amount of weight from fat one loses may be equal to the amount of weight gained from increased muscle. Or the muscle weight may even exceed the fat weight lost as muscle weighs more than fat. Weighing yourself under these circumstances will not tell you if you are losing fat. Instead have your percent body fat estimated at about eight-week intervals to see if you are losing body fat and take body measurements to see if you are slimming down. Inches may come off even when pounds don't. You can actually lose fat, gain weight, and look better all at the same time.

Women:	Date:_____	Date:_____	Date:_____
Calf:	R_____ L_____	R_____ L_____	R_____ L_____
Thigh:	R_____ L_____	R_____ L_____	R_____ L_____
Buttocks:	R_____ L_____	R_____ L_____	R_____ L_____
Hips:	_____	_____	_____

Waist:						
Chest:						
Upper Arm:	R _____ L _____		R _____ L _____		R _____ L _____	

Men:	Date:_____		Date:_____		Date:_____	
Calf:	R _____ L _____		R _____ L _____		R _____ L _____	
Thigh:	R _____ L _____		R _____ L _____		R _____ L _____	
Buttocks:	R _____ L _____		R _____ L _____		R _____ L _____	
Abdomen:	_____		_____		_____	
Chest′ (relaxed):	_____		_____		_____	
Chest (expanded):	_____		_____		_____	
Upper Arm (relaxed):	R _____ L _____		R _____ L _____		R _____ L _____	
Upper Arm (flexed):	R _____ L _____		R _____ L _____		R _____ L _____	
Shoulders:	_____		_____		_____	
Neck (optional):	_____		_____		_____	

Activity 2: Can this body be saved?

Scenario #1:
Kelly is a 19-year-old college freshman. She is 5'4", weighs 144 pounds and has 29 percent body fat. Ever since she can remember, she has always been a little overweight. Every member of her family is also overweight. "My mother has always been a good cook, and much of our family and social lives resolve around preparing and eating food. I have just accepted the fact that I will always be overweight."

Most likely, Kelly is a precontemplator and does not think about losing weight. What suggestions can you make for her which will help her move to the contemplator stage?

Scenario #2

By age 25, Cory's life had changed. Marriage, children, graduation, and a new job had placed new demands on his time and energy. Like many young fathers, his new life had taken a toll on his once strong lean body. He had become fat and out of shape. His percent body fat had increased from a healthy 17 percent to an all-time high of 24 percent. Cory says his problem is his lack of time. He wants to lose weight but just doesn't have the same amount of free time he used to have.

Cory is a contemplator who can't overcome some of his weight loss barriers. What are his barriers and how can he overcome them?

What about diet? How can he use diet to ensure weight loss and weight loss maintenance?

Activity 3: Self quiz on safe and effective weight-loss strategies.

From the following list of features taken from real diets, mark those you think are part of a safe and effective diet. Check your answers in the key below.

_____ 1. Eat as much food as you like, as long as your diet includes lots of fruit.

_____ 2. Eat normally for four days, followed by four days of eating just grapefruit.

_____ 3. Jog seven days a week for an hour each time.

_____ 4. No need to exercise.

_____ 5. Set goals, plan rewards, and develop social support activities.

_____ 6. Eat meals that consist of 75 percent protein.

_____ 7. Expend more energy than you consume.

_____ 8. Take an appetite suppressant before each meal.

_____ 9. Perform endurance-type exercise three days a week.

_____ 10. Consume no fewer than 900 calories a day.

Note: Items five, seven and nine are known to be safe and effective.

LABS

Lab 8.1 What Can I Do? (pages 207–208)
Lab 8.2 Calculating Daily Caloric Expenditure (pages 209–210)

ADDITIONAL INFORMATION

Adiposity

Fat cells are also called adipose cells. The term adiposity refers to the number and size of fat cells, which is largely determined by genetics and the amount and type of food we consume. Fat cells are produced throughout the first few years of life and during adolescence. Once a fat cell is produced it remains in the body for life.

The amount of fat in the cell can vary according to the amount of excess energy a person consumes. In lean individuals, most fat cells contain very little fat; in the obese, fat cells are usually full of fat. The enlargement of a fat cell is known as hypertrophy. It is believed that fat cells can store limited amounts of fat before they divide into two separate cells in a process called hyperplasia. This occurs when fat cells have exceeded their fat-storing capacity. Hyperplasia is thought to be common among obese people and infants. Researchers even suggest that overfeeding during infancy leads to the creation of new fat cells, which may increase a person's chance of being overweight or obese as an adult. The number of fat cells in obese children is often three times that in normal weight children, which often leads to obesity as adults.

Obese adults have more and larger fat cells than do normal weight individuals. Body fat that is stored in fat cells created through hyperplasia is difficult to lose. All fat cells retain a minimum amount of fat at all time, and total body fat is closely related to the total number of fat cells a person may have. The longer one remains obese, the more difficult it is to remove extra fat because the cells have grown accustomed to having it. This phenomenon helps explain why the body tries to retain a certain body weight, as described by the set point theory discussed earlier in this chapter.

Spot Reducing

Perhaps one of the biggest all-time diet and exercise myths is spot reducing. Countless gimmicks have been developed to exercise a specific part of your body, with the promise that fat stored in that part of the body will disappear. You cannot choose where the fat will come off. In general, it will come off gradually all over. If fat tends to accumulate in one place on your body, you can speculate with some certainty that where it went on first, it will come off last. Don't fall into the trap of thinking that because you use your legs to run, you will get rid of the fat on your thighs more quickly. Running on your hands could be just as effective on leg fat. Of course, running on your legs will tone up the leg muscles underneath the fat, and running on your hand, if that were possible or practical, would certainly help tone your arms and improve your balance!

RESOURCES

Suggested Reading

Bennion, L.J., E.L. Bierman, J.M. Ferguson, and the Editors of Consumer Reports Books. *Straight talk about weight control: Taking the pounds off and keeping them off.* Yonkers, NY: Consumers Union, 1991.

Gilbert, S. *The Psychology of Dieting.* New York: Rutledge, 1989.

Grodner, M. Forever dieting: A chronic dieting syndrome. *Journal of Nutrition Education* 24(4):207-11. 1992.

Kano, S. *Making peace with food*. New York: Harper & Row, 1989.

Ornish, D. *Eat more, weigh less: Dr. Dean Ornish's life choice program for losing weight safely while eating abundantly*. New York: HarperCollins, 1993.

Organizations

Overeaters Anonymous General Services Office
P.O. Box 4305
San Pedro, CA 90732

Overeaters Anonymous World Services
6075 Zenith Court, NE
Rio Rancho, NM 87124
Web site: www.overeatersanonymous.org
www.overeaters.org

National Association of Anorexia Nervosa and
Associated Disorders
Box 7
Highland Park, IL 60035

National Eating Disorders Organization (NEDO)
6655 South Yale Avenue
Tulsa, OK 74136
Tel: (918) 481-4044
Fax: (918) 481-4076
Web site: www.laureate.com/nedo

YMCA of the USA
101 North Wacker Drive
Chicago, IL 60606
Tel: (312) 977-0031
Fax: (312) 977-9063
Web site: www.ymca.net

YWCA of the USA
Empire State Building
Suite 301
New York, NY 10118
Tel: (212) 275-0800
Fax: (21) 465-2281
Web site: www.ywca.org

Videos

How Healthy is your Diet? YMCA Program Store.
Box 5077, Champaign, IL 61820.

Life in the Fat Lane. A documentary featuring Connie Chung. Dealing with the problems associated with obesity and eating disorders. Available from NBC Television.

Preventing Cardiovascular Disease

Chapter 9

CHAPTER SUMMARY

Even though cardiovascular disease is the leading cause of death for half of all Americans, very few young adults experience the disease. For many, the disease is something you get when you are older. Heart disease is the most preventable of all the major causes of death, but prevention must begin early in life to be effective. College age students are ideally positioned to prevent this disease. Making good choices about the use of tobacco, exercise, and dietary habits can all help in prevention. Treatment for cardiovascular diseases also includes lifestyle changes so it makes sense to adopt good habits early in life and limit the chance of ever having to experience disease.

LEARNING OBJECTIVES

The student will be able to:
- describe the trend in the prevalence of cardiovascular disease since 1950.
- describe the most common forms of cardiovascular diseases.
- describe how arteriosclerosis (atherosclerosis) develops.
- list and explain the difference between the modifiable and nonmodifiable risk factors of cardiovascular disease.
- explain the dangers of each modifiable risk factor and discuss how each risk factor can be reduced.
- explain the role lifestyle plays in the prevention and treatment of cardiovascular disease.
- list the common warning signs of a heart attack.
- list the common warning signs of a stroke.
- describe four ways to diagnose heart disease.
- describe four ways to treat heart disease.

PERSONAL PROFILE

Doug Stone: Singing a New Tune

Who would have imagined that it was possible to have a heart attack and undergo quadruple bypass surgery before the age of 36, yet that's what happened to Doug Stone, one of the most popular country music stars of the 90's. Doug was as surprised as anyone. "I didn't think I had a heart problem at 35," he said, "but every time I started walking, my chest would hurt." After his first medical examination failed to identify the partially blocked arteries that supplied most of his heart's blood. Stone went back on tour doing what he loved most, making country music.

His stellar music career includes several albums, five Top 5 country hits, and hundreds of performances across the nation. After a few months, however, his condition worsened, and when he could no longer take the pain, he returned to the Centennial Medical Center in Nashville. His 29-year-old wife, Carie, recalls, "When they told me a quadruple bypass, I almost fell over." The cardiologist who diagnosed Stone's condition showed them that one of the main arteries of his heart was 99 percent closed. In the doctor's own words, "He was a heart attack waiting to happen."

How could so much artery damage happen in a person so young? Early in his life. Stone started living a lifestyle that can eventually end with heart disease. Childhood in a broken home and little parental guidance eventually resulted in his dropping out of school, early marriage, and raising two children while working as a mechanic. When his first marriage ended in divorce and he lost custody of his two children, he entered a three-year battle with depression. This dark period of his life ended when he remarried. Perhaps the biggest cause of his heart condition was his well-established addiction to fried foods and three packs of cigarettes a day. The cumulative affect of tobacco use, high-fat foods, stress, and lack of exercise had finally resulted in a life-or-death situation.

Five weeks after the operation, Stone was back making music, but things are different. A large vegetable garden near his home supplies much of his low-fat cholesterol diet while a Stairstepper and rowing machine take up a large part of the livingroom. "Life," concedes Carie, who admits she waits anxiously for her husband's daily phone calls from the road, "will never be quite the same."

Adapted from Dougherty, S. and D. Carlisle, This heart of Stone's, *People Weekly* 38:96-98, July 20, 1992.

CONTENT OUTLINE

I.   Cardiovascular disease (CVD) is the number one cause of death among American adults.
- A.   It kills five times the number of people who die of lung or breast cancer and is responsible for almost half of all deaths.
- B.   The best prevention is a healthy lifestyle starting early in life.
- C.   CVD includes more than 20 different diseases that affect the heart and vessels of the body.
- D.   The most common diseases are:
  - 1.   coronary heart disease
  - 2.   stroke
  - 3.   hypertension
- E.   Modifiable risk factors include:
  - 1.   diet
  - 2.   stress
  - 3.   high blood cholesterol
  - 4.   smoking
  - 5.   inactivity
- F.   Nonmodifiable risk factors include:
  - 1.   age
  - 2.   gender
  - 3.   race

           4.   heredity

II.   Cardiovascular diseases: past and present trends

    A.   CVD starts early in life even though the effects may not be felt for many years.
        1.   1953 research study on Korean soldiers killed in combat with an average age of 22 years revealed that 77 % of the 300 soldiers showed advanced levels of blood vessel blockage

    B.   One hundred fifteen (115) million Americans are living with CVD.

    C.   Society's cost for CVD is over $135 billion dollars in medical expenses.

    D.   Prevalence of heart disease has been cut in half since the 1950's and is still dropping.
        1.   hailed as one of the greatest public health accomplishments in this century
        2.   reductions have included men and women of all races

    E.   Lifestyle changes are largely responsible for the reduction in heart disease.
        1.   fewer people smoke
        2.   more people try to control their cholesterol and blood pressure
        3.   more people make exercise part of their daily lives

    F.   Improved medical treatments and facilities have also reduced the number of cases of heart disease.

III.   Types of CVD

    A.   Arteriosclerosis is any arterial disease that leads to thickening and hardening of the arteries.
        1.   atherosclerosis is the most common form of arteriosclerosis
            a.   consists of an accumulation of plaque in the arteries, which narrows the vessel
            b.   plaque deposits can range from small streaks to large lesions
            c.   process is widespread throughout the population and appears to begin early in life
        2.   when the arteries that supply the heart are narrowed, the heart's blood supply is reduced and ischemia results
        3.   resulting oxygen starvation causes severe chest pain, called angina pectoris
            a.   angina can often be detected by participating in a maximum endurance test

    B.   Myocardial infarction or heart attack, is caused by a blocked coronary artery.
        1.   artery may become blocked by a blood clot, or by gradual narrowing of the artery
            a.   warning signs of a heart attack:
                (1)   chest discomfort with light-headedness, fainting, sweating, nausea, or shortness of breath.
                (2)   pain that spreads to the shoulders, neck, or arms.
                (3)   an uncomfortable pressure, fullness, squeezing, or pain in the center of the chest that lasts more than a few minutes or goes away and returns.
            b.   each year 350,000 Americans die from heart attacks before reaching the hospital.

    C.   Stroke is a form of CVD that affects the vessels that supply blood to the brain (cerebral arteries).
        1.   most common cause of stroke is a thrombosis, or blood clot, which forms in the arteries of the brain
        2.   some strokes are caused by an aneurysm or a weakened section of the artery that expands until it bursts

3.　one third of all stroke victims die, one-third are permanently disabled, and one-third gradually return to an acceptable quality of life

4.　the most common risk factor is hypertension

5.　stroke warning signs are:

   a.　sudden weakness or numbness on one side of the face, arm, or leg.

   b.　temporary loss of speech or vision, unexplained dizziness, or headache.

6.　drugs are used to dissolve the blood clot in the arteries for heart attack and stroke victims.

   a.　the sooner the stroke patient gets a drug to dissolve the blood clot, the less damage is likely

   b.　drugs must be given within three to six hours after the signs of a stroke start.

7.　Hypertension is when blood pressure is chronically elevated.

   a.　the most common type of vascular disease

   b.　25 percent of the United States population is affected.

   c.　may be related to other body organ problems, such as kidney, liver

   d.　several factors have been linked to the occurrence of hypertension: age, African American heritage, obesity, heredity, sodium sensitivity, lack of exercise, and excessive alcohol consumption.

IV.　Modifiable risk factors

  A.　Inactivity (sedentary living)

    1.　inactivity is one of the best predictors of CVD

    2.　cardiovascular disease is associated with low levels of cardiovascular endurance

      a.　in 1991, a national survey reported 58.1 percent of adults report irregular or no physical activity.

    3.　individuals who expended 2,000 calories of energy per week in physical activity had the greatest reduction in the incidence of heart disease.

      a.　to expend 2,000 calories per week, the average adult would have to walk briskly for 4.77 hours or jog for two hours

        (1)　the important conclusion is that doing any type of physical activity can help reduce a person's risk of heart disease

  B.　Cigarette smoking

    1.　the number one risk factor associated with death in the United States

    2.　responsible for more deaths from CVD than deaths due to cancer

      a.　nicotine

        (1)　increases heart rate.

        (2)　affects blood lipid by increasing LDL levels and decrease HDLs

      b.　carbon monoxide in tobacco smokes displaces oxygen in the blood.

      c.　constricted blood vessels, reduced oxygen in arterial blood, and higher levels of blood pressure all cause the heart to work harder and can produce cardiac arrhythmias that can lead to cardiac arrest.

    3.　secondhand smoking (environmental tobacco smoke, passive smoking), which is inhaling other people's tobacco smoke, increases risk of CVD

      a.　 nonsmoking spouses of smokers are 3 times more likely to die of a heart attack than those married to nonsmokers

      b.　children of smokers have a high rate of bronchitis, asthma, and other respiratory disorders

C.   Chronic high levels of stress
1. individuals who are depressed, stressed, or overly anxious have an increased incidence of cardiovascular disease.
2. stress increases blood pressure, heart rate, and the number of fatty acids released into the blood
3. associated with higher levels of blood cholesterol and blood pressure

D.   Obesity (excessive body fat)
1. can elevate levels of blood cholesterol and blood pressure
2. regular aerobic exercise and dietary intervention will help lose body fat and reduce the risk of heart disease

E.   Cholesterol
1. long-term studies link it to heart disease
2. substance found only in animal tissues
3. needed to:
   a. build cell membranes
   b. produce hormones for the development of sex characteristics
   c. help digest fat
   d. properly develop the young nervous system
4. combined with lipoprotein in order to make it water-soluble so it can travel through the blood stream
   a. a thick protein shell around the cholesterol makes high-density lipoproteins or HDLs
   b. a thinner protein shell around the cholesterol makes low-density lipoproteins or LDLs
5. HDL—the "good cholesterol"
   a. picks up cholesterol from the blood and tissues and delivers it to the liver where it is converted to bile and used for digestion or disposed of
   b. high levels of HDL help remove cholesterol from the arterial walls and blood, reducing arterial plaque and risk of CVD
   c. average HDL values are 45 mg/dl for men and 55 mg/dl for women
      (1) $\geq$ 45 mg/dl is considered desirable
   d. HDL levels can be increased with:
      (1) regular moderate to vigorous aerobic exercise
      (2) weight loss
   e. HDL levels can decrease if a person is:
      (1) overweight
      (2) smoking or chewing tobacco
      (3) using steroids
      (4) medical condition like diabetes
6. LDL—the "bad cholesterol"
   a. LDLs release and deposit cholesterol to body cells including vessel walls
   b. liver has sites for LDL but when LDL levels are high the sites are full and excess LDLs are free to deposit cholesterol elsewhere
   c. LDL can be lowered through:
      (1) regular exercise

                    (2)   a diet low in saturated fat
                    (3)   weight loss
                    (4)   medication
        d.   LDL levels below 130 mg/dl are desirable

7. Total Cholesterol
    a.   sum of HDL and LDL
    b.   below 200 mg/dl is desirable with HDL above 35 mg/dl
    c.   in a study of 4,000 men with high cholesterol, a 25 % decrease in cholesterol resulted in 50 % fewer heart attacks
    d.   for every 1 % of cholesterol lost there is a corresponding 2% decrease in heart disease risk

8. sources of cholesterol
    a.   diet
            (1)   average consumption is 500–600 mg daily
            (2)   recommended consumption is 300 mg daily
            (3)   found only in animal foods (meat and dairy products)
    b.   body
            (1)   cholesterol is produced by the liver
            (2)   produces 1,000–2,000 mg daily
            (3)   produces more cholesterol when saturated fat is available
            (4)   when less saturated fat is consumed. cholesterol production is reduced

9. cholesterol reduction
    a.   diet high in fiber and low in fat (especially saturated fat)
            (1)   fiber may combine with cholesterol and help prevent absorption during digestion
            (2)   diet high in fiber is naturally low in fat
    b.   regular aerobic exercise and weight loss
            (1)   since weight loss is usually coupled with exercise, researchers are unclear as to whether the exercise, the weight loss or both are affecting blood cholesterol levels
    c.   reduction in stress
    d.   smoking cessation

F.   High blood pressure
    1.   blood pressure is the force exerted against vessel walls as blood moves through them with the pumping of the heart
    2.   high blood pressure occurs when the vessel walls exert too much tension on the blood flowing through them
    3.   often called "the silent killer." hypertension often does not produce outward symptoms or signs
    4.   over the years hypertension can quietly damage blood vessels and some organs
    5.   measured and recorded as a fraction with systolic pressure on top and diastolic pressure on the bottom
        a.   systolic pressure is the pressure in the vessels when the heart is pushing blood out into the blood vessels
        b.   diastolic pressure is the pressure in the vessels between heart beats
        c.   systolic pressures over 140 mmHg are considered elevated

        d.   diastolic pressures over 90 mmHg are considered elevated

        e.   to be diagnosed with high blood pressure a person must exhibit a blood pressure above 140/90 mmHg on several occasions (see Table 9.2)

6.   high blood pressure is dangerous

        a.   prolonged hypertension causes the smooth middle lining of arteries to lose their elasticity and become hardened and rigid which then forces the heart to pump harder to move blood through the arteries

        b.   heart enlarges (bigger muscle needed to pump harder) but becomes constrained by the sac surrounding the heart, making it less efficient

        c.   atherosclerosis accelerates when hypertension and high blood cholesterol are both present, which can lead to:

            (1)   blocked arteries in the heart (heart attack)

            (2)   blocked arteries in the brain (stroke)

            (3)   kidney, liver and eye damage

7.   controlling high blood pressure

        a.   lose excess body weight

            (1)   most effective method of lowering blood pressure

            (2)   excess body fat can cause a two- to six-fold increase in the risk of hypertension

            (3)   fat loss can lead to a decrease in both systolic and diastolic pressures

        b.   reduce sodium intake

            (1)   recommended consumption is 2.5 grams

                (a)   one teaspoon of salt contains 2.5 grams sodium

                (b)   average intake is 2–4 times higher

                (c)   reduction of one-half teaspoon has been shown to reduce systolic pressure by 5 mmHg and diastolic pressure by 2.5 mmHg

            (2)   if everyone reduces salt to recommended intake, then those who are sensitive to salt will be prevented from having high blood pressure

            (3)   tips for reducing salt

                (a)   limit the use of foods with visible salt (pretzels, etc.)

                (b)   choose more fruits and vegetables

                (c)   substitute salt with other herbs when cooking

                (d)   read food labels and avoid high sodium foods

                (e)   don't add salt to processed foods

        c.   limit alcohol consumption

            (1)   regular consumption of 3–4 drinks a day increases blood pressure

            (2)   heavy drinkers have 4 times the risk of being hypertensive

            (3)   some studies show that fewer than 2 drinks per day reduces heart disease risk

                (a)   alcohol may reduce the blood's ability to clot and may increase HDLs when consumed in moderate amounts

                (b)   medical community does not recommend drinking alcohol as a treatment for hypertension, as the cure may cause more damage than the disease

      d.   exercise
- (1) contracting and expanding of smooth arterial muscle during exercise is beneficial in reducing blood pressure
- (2) immediately after exercise, blood pressure is usually 10–20 mmHg lower than before exercise
  - (a) this effect lasts for 20 minutes to 2 hours
- (3) researchers believe that a physically active lifestyle can reduce systolic and diastolic pressures by 10 mmHg
  - (a) effect with 20 minutes of endurance activity 3–5 times per week at 40–60 % of maximum oxygen uptake
  - (b) resistance exercise raises blood pressure during the activity and does not reduce blood pressure afterward

      e.   treat with medication
- (1) only after lifestyle interventions are insufficient
- (2) medication treats symptoms, not the cause
- (3) only one in five persons on medication manages to reduce their blood pressure below 140/90 mmHg
- (4) side effects include weakness, leg cramps, stuffy nose, diarrhea, impotence, and skin rash

V.   Nonmodifiable risk factors

    A.   Age
1. one out of every two deaths after the age of 65 are caused by CVD.
2. age greater than 65 is associated with 80 percent of all fatal heart attacks.
3. older people who don't smoke , have safe levels of blood pressure and cholesterol, and eat a proper diet decrease their risk of CVD.

    B.   Heredity
1. a family history of heart disease is the best predictor of heart disease.
2. people with a biologically related relative who had heart disease before age 65 are considered to have a family history of heart disease.
3. one study showed that people with a known history of heart disease also have high blood pressure, a second major risk factor.

    C.   Race
1. African American males have an increased risk of stroke and CVD, primarily owing to high rates of hypertension.
2. 33 percent of African American males are hypertensive, compared with 11 percent of the general population.
3. African American females do not have the same hypertension rate; they do have a high level of obesity. 50 percent of all African American women are overweight compared to 32 percent of African American males and 33 percent of the general population.

    D.   Gender
1. women do not have the same risk of CVD as do men
2. estrogen provides some level of protection to women
   - a. estrogen helps keep cholesterol low which helps prevent atherosclerosis
   - b. hormone replacement therapy can reduce risk due to lack of estrogen

        3.   by age 65 women have substantially higher rates of CVD, but still lower than men

VI.   Reversing CVD—using the same lifestyle habits that prevent it

    A.   Studies have demonstrated that drug and diet therapy can lower LDLs and raise HDLs with the effect of retarding progression of artery plaque and promoting plaque regression.

    B.   Studies involving medication, diet, and lifestyle intervention have demonstrated dramatic regressions of arterial disease and 50% fewer cardiovascular events (heart attacks, death etc.).

    C.   Most studies so far have used drastic interventions (e.g. a diet with only 10% fat) over short periods of time.

VII.   Diagnosing CVD involves regular medical examinations which may include a(n):

    A.   Electrocardiogram (ECG)

        1.   monitors the electrical activity of the heart; look for abnormal electrical patterns in the ECG printout

        2.   resting ECG (lying down) may or may not pick up heart problems

        3.   treadmill (or cycle) stress test is more apt to pick up heart problems

            a.   person jogs, walks, or rides a bicycle ergometer at increasingly more difficult levels while the heart is monitored

            b.   heart problems will usually surface at peak performance exertion levels

    B.   Thallium test

        1.   radioactive thallium is injected into the bloodstream during the last minute of a treadmill test

        2.   radioactive-sensitive sensors create a 3-dimensional picture of the heart and arteries and illuminate any blockage problems that exist

    C.   Echocardiogram uses sound waves to produce a 3-dimensional picture which allows doctors to measure heart size, heart wall thickness, and check heart valve function

VIII.   Treating CVD

    A.   Medications

        1.   lower blood pressure

        2.   lower blood cholesterol

        3.   control abnormal heart rhythms

        4.   relieve angina pain

        5.   reduce the seriousness of heart attacks

            b.   anti-clotting drugs (clot-busters) dissolve clots that may be blocking arteries

            c.   most effective in the early stages of a heart attack

    B.   Balloon angioplasty (percutaneous transluminal coronary angioplasty or PTCA)

        1.   a balloon-tipped catheter is inserted into the artery, the balloon is inflated, causing the blockage to be smashed and the plaque cracked

    C.   Coronary artery bypass

        1.   surgical attachment of a length of leg vein to the aorta and to the blocked artery below the blockage

    D.   Heart transplant

        1.   the heart of the patient is replaced with a donor heart from a cadaver

        2.   65 percent of heart transplant patients are alive after 5 years

BEHAVIOR BOOSTS: STAGE-BASED STUDENT ACTIVITIES

Precontemplator
- Consider getting your cholesterol checked to determine whether you are at risk.
- Find out whether your family is prone to heart disease (Ask yourself if any of your grandparents, parents, or brothers or sisters have had heart disease).
- Talk to friends or relatives who have had heart disease and ask if they would do anything differently if they were thirty years younger.
- Ask one or both of your parents to take the survey in lab 9.2 and then compare your scores.

Contemplator
- Visit with someone who has heart disease. Ask how life has changed since they were diagnosed with the disease.
- Brainstorm alone or with a friend about behaviors that would lower your risk of heart disease.
- Consider how a person's quality of life can be changed by heart disease.

Preparer
- List three small things you can do today to lower your risk of heart disease. Try doing one of them each day for a week.
- Write one short-term goal to reduce your risk of heart disease.
- Try substituting a low-fat food for a high-fat one.
- Refer to chapters 3 and 6 for ideas on changing your exercise and diet habits.
- Have your blood pressure and cholesterol checked this week.
- Exercise today.

Action Taker
- Name something or someone that is supporting your new behaviors.
- What is the most tempting situation you face with your new behavior? How do you withstand it?
- Identify the things you're doing to prevent CVD and try one additional preventative measure from the following: exercise regularly, don't smoke, eat a low fat diet, keep stress under control, have ideal body weight, have acceptable cholesterol and blood pressure.

Maintainer
- Keep your own log of your blood pressure and cholesterol levels.
- Make a list of the rewards you get by practicing behaviors that lower your risk of heart disease.
- Talk with a friend about the importance of preventing CVD.

ADDITIONAL SUGGESTED STUDENT ACTIVITIES

Activity 1: Monitoring Blood Pressure

Follow the directions in Activity 9.1 on page 222 and the chart on page 220.
If your blood pressure is high, consider ways to bring it down and discuss these with your physician.

Activity 2: Monitoring Cholesterol

Have your cholesterol checked by a trained professional. Refer to the chart on page 219.
If your cholesterol is high, consider ways to bring it down and discuss these with your physician.

Activity 3: Substituting Healthy Foods

Have students list some of the "bad" foods in their diet. Then have them try to name a healthy food they could substitute for the "bad" food. After attempting to do this, refer students to the informational box on page 224.

Activity 4: Cardiac Rehabilitation

Visit a cardiac rehabilitation center. Learn how people are encouraged to diet and exercise following a heart attack. Talk with individuals concerning their motivation to change before and after the incident. Discuss adherence to the program with members and the director. Watch an exercise stress test.

Activity 5: Bypass Surgery

Watch bypass surgery on video/film or live at a hospital.

LABS

Lab 9.1 What Can I Do? (pages 227–228)
Lab 9.2 Assessing Heart Disease Risk (pages 229–230)

RESOURCES

Suggested Reading

American Heart Association. *Heart and stroke facts*. Dallas, TX, 1995.

Bouchard, C., R.J. Shepard, T. Stephens, J.R. Sutton, and B.D. McPherson. *Exercise, Fitness and Health: A Consensus of Current Knowledge*. Champaign, IL: Human Kinetics , 1990

Donatelle, R. and L. Davis. *Access to Health*. Englewood Cliffs, NJ: Prentice Hall, 1993.

Editors of Consumer Guide. *Cholesterol: Your guide for a healthy heart*. Lincolnwood, IL: Publications International, 1994.

Fischman, J. Type A on trial. *Psychology Today*. February, 1987.

Fox, S.I. *Human Physiology*. Dubuque, IA: W.C. Brown, 1996.

Hamann, B. *Disease: Identification, prevention, and control*, St. Louis: Mosby, 1994.

Lorig, K., D. Laurent, H.Holman, V. Gonzalez, D. Sobel, and M. Minior. *Living a healthy life with chronic conditions*. Palo Alto, CA: Bull Publishing, 1994.

Organizations

American Heart Association
National Center
7272 Greenville Avenue
Dallas, TX 75231
Tel (800) AHA-USA1 (Customer Heart & Stroke Information)
Tel (888) MY-HEART (Women's Health Information)
Web site: http://www.aha.org

National Heart, Lung and Blood Institute
Department of Health and Human Services
Building 31, Room 4A-21
9000 Rockville Pike
Bethesda, MD 20205
Tel: (301) 496-4236

Additional Local and Community Resources

American Red Cross
Hospitals
Cardiac Rehabilitation Centers

Cancer and Other Common Threats to Wellness

Chapter 10

CHAPTER SUMMARY

Cancer is the second leading cause of death in the United States. Like heart disease, it is caused by several factors, the most important of which may be lifestyle. Of the various forms of cancer, lung cancer is the most common and the most preventable. Tobacco use is the primary cause of this disease. Other forms of cancer may not be as easily prevented, but many can be detected early enough to increase one's chances of a complete recovery. A wellness lifestyle uses diet and exercise to reduce the risk of many cancers. It also employs the use of early detection practices such as breast or testicular self-examination. Other common ailments such as diabetes, headaches, allergies, and asthma may not be completely preventable, but they are treatable. Knowing how to recognize these conditions and how to treat them can add significantly to a person's quality of life.

LEARNING OBJECTIVES

The student will be able to:
- define cancer and discuss the theories regarding how cancer develops.
- list the major risk factors and causes for the most common forms of cancer.
- describe prevention measures for cancer.
- explain the role of exercise as it concerns cancer prevention.
- explain the role of diet as it concerns cancer prevention.
- describe how the most common cancers are detected and treated including radiation, chemotherapy, and immunotherapy.
- determine which lifestyle habits should be changed and/or maintained to prevent cancer.
- describe both types of diabetes mellitus.
- discuss the management of diabetes mellitus through medication and exercise.
- explain the sources for, methods to prevent, and ways to alleviate three types of headaches.
- explain the allergic response and identify common triggers.
- describe asthma.
- list common triggers for asthma attacks.
- discuss the management of asthma including exercise-induced asthma.

PERSONAL PROFILE

George Sheehan: Finishing Life With Wellness

George Sheehan was a cardiologist, runner, philosopher, father, writer, and speaker. In November, 1993, he died of prostate cancer. George was known as the American guru of running. During his seventy-five years of life, he influenced Americans in such a way that running was transformed from a casual pastime to a national craze. In addition to completing hundreds of races and setting world records, George was a practicing cardiologist, father of twelve children, and author of several best-selling books. Through his books and speeches, he shared the benefits and joys of running with millions of people. Whatever he did, he did well.

Much of life changed in 1986 when he was diagnosed with inoperable prostate cancer. At that point, the cancer had spread to his bones and his doctors gave him only a few years. "When I first found out about the cancer, I lay awake at night," he said. "I couldn't go to sleep. You really panic when you first get it. The first thing you do is try to bargain your way out of it. We say, I'll be good from now on if only I can get off the hook and live longer. Then you start thinking about a cure. I went to Detroit and the National Institutes of Health before I finally realized that no matter what they gave me, the chance for a cure was slim. At that point, I began to accept what was happening to me."

Not everyone was born to be a runner, and not everyone will be an athlete, but without exception, all of us will die. When faced with terminal illness, many people pause to reevaluate their lives. George best summed up his feelings when he said, "So much of life passes without our being in it all." Cancer forced him to count every day and make the most of what was truly important in his life.

Cancer victims realize that life is too short to get caught up in an endless cycle of self-centered pursuits. Many have said that when face-to-face with their own mortality, worldly possessions and accomplishments become irrelevant and the only things of importance are family and friends. George came to the same conclusion while he still had time to make a difference. Before his death, he was able to spend his remaining years patching up his family relationships and loving his children and grandchildren. By his own confession he became much less self-absorbed. Most likely, if he had his life to live all over again, he would re-focus his efforts on the truly important things in life: family and friends.

Adapted from Henderson, J. There is no finish line. *Runners World*, 30(3):18, 1995, and Burfoot, A. A tribute to George Sheehan: just call me George. *Runners World*, 29(Jan):54-56, 1994.

CONTENT OUTLINE

I. Cancer is a prevalent disease for which risk can be reduced through healthy lifestyle habits.
    A. Statistics from the U.S. Department of Health and Human Services
        1. the number two cause of death in the U.S.
        2. one out of every three people will eventually have some form of cancer
        3. responsible for one out of every five deaths in U.S.
    B. With the exception of lung cancer, the number of cases of other cancers is either remaining the same or decreasing. Lung cancer will likely decrease in the future as a reflection of fewer smokers.
    C. Lung, colorectal (colon & rectal), and breast cancer together represent more than half the cases of cancer.

    D.   The average survival time for cancer victims is increasing.
        1.   white patients have a 50 % chance of survival, African Americans only 37%
            a.   differences are in part due to socioeconomic issues like access to health care
        2.   early detection and improved treatments have helped survival

II.   Cancer is a group of over 100 different diseases characterized by the uncontrolled growth and spread of abnormal cells.
    A.   When a normal cell undergoes an abnormal change, a mutated cell is produced.
        1.   normal cells multiply in an orderly fashion, replacing old or injured cells or building new tissue
    B.   Abnormal cells do not grow in an orderly way; they grow and multiply in a random fashion, developing into clusters of abnormal cells called tumors.
    C.   Tumors can be benign or malignant.
        1.   Benign tumors tend to stay confined to a space, don't spread, and aren't life threatening. Only dangerous if they crowd other organs and interfere with function.
        2.   Malignant tumors are made up of cancerous cells.
            a.   very dangerous if not detected early, damage tissues
            b.   can spread (metastasize) to surrounding tissue or invade other tissues by traveling through the bloodstream and lymphatic system
            c.   microscopic examination of tissue is required to determine malignancy

III.   Cancer theories
    A.   Spontaneous error occurs during cell reproduction.
        1.   genetic errors may be caused by cells that are older or that have been exposed to stress or injury
        2.   the genetic sequence of the parent cell is broken or changed and that change is passed on to all cells created from the parent cell
    B.   Cancer-causing genes called oncogenes are activated.
        1.   all chromosomes have a few genes, called oncogenes, that may be cancer-causing but which are usually dormant
        2.   oncogenes may be activated by some external agent or condition such as age, stress, toxins, radiation, viruses, sunshine
        3.   researchers are unclear whether oncogenes are inherited or whether they are normal genes that are somehow altered
    C.   The alteration of normal genes into cancer-causing genes by the effects of certain external agents or substances that enter the cell and cause the genetic sequencing of the cell to be altered.
        1.   probably most widely believed cancer theory
        2.   cancer-causing agents are called carcinogens
        3.   researchers have a hard time "proving" something is cancer-causing

IV.   Causes of cancer
    A.   Heredity
        1.   family histories of cancer suggest a genetic link but could also be a shared environment, lifestyle, or exposure to radiation, etc.
        2.   abnormal gene sequences that relate to some forms of cancer have been found but just because a person has a defective sequence does not mean s/he will develop cancer
        3.   number of cases thought to be caused by genetics is very small
    B.   Race (inherited factor)

           1.   death rates from cancer from highest to lowest are: Black males, White males, Black women, White women, Asian, Hispanic and American Indian males, American Indian, Hispanic, and Asian women.

           2.   race is related to cancer but is not a cause of cancer

           3.   differences in rates between races probably due to education, access to quality medical care, diet or other social and cultural difference

C.   Gender (inherited factor)

           1.   certain cancers are more prevalent in one gender but can occur in both (e.g., breast cancer)

           2.   some cancers are gender specific such as prostate and uterine cancer

D.   Environment

           1.   perhaps the biggest cause of cancer

           2.   occupational hazards include: asbestos exposure, coal dust, inhalants and solvents used for painting and auto repair, herbicides and pesticides, etc.

           3.   home hazards include: asbestos exposure, water born carcinogens, second hand smoke, radon etc.

E.   Food additives

           1.   Food and Drug Administration (FDA) does extensive research before an additive is permitted in food.

           2.   FDA gave approval for saccharin but only with a warning label that it may have cancer-causing effects. The American Diabetic Association feels that the cancer-causing effects that might be associated with saccharin are outweighed by the risks of diabetics failing to maintain proper blood sugar.

           3.   some evidence linking nitrates to esophageal and stomach cancer (nitrates are used to smoke or cure meats like bacon, sausage, and other dried meats)

F.   Cigarette smoke

           1.   causes the greatest number of cancer cases and is the most preventable

           2.   is the number one cause of lung cancer

           3.   breathing second hand smoke increases cancer risk

           4.   babies born to smoking women or women who live in second hand smoke environments had traces of smoke-related chemicals in their hair

G.   Radiation

           1.   exposure to radioactive substances increases risk of cancer

           2.   ultraviolet light is a form of radiation

                a.   there are 600,000 cases of skin cancer yearly

                b.   most skin cancer is treated and cured by burning off or surgically removing the abnormal cells

                c.   4–5 % of skin cancers are serious enough to be potentially fatal

H.   Viruses

           1.   leukemia, lymphomas, and cancers of the liver and cervix can be caused by viruses

                a.   viruses will not usually cause cancer unless the immune system is also compromised

                b.   herpes virus can cause leukemia

                c.   human immunodeficiency virus (HIV) can lead to some cancers

V.   Types of cancer: categorized according to the type of body tissue they affect

    A.   Carcinomas: found in epithelial tissues (tissues that line the body surfaces or cavities)

        1.   account for most forms of cancer

        2.   breast, skin, lung, intestinal, pancreatic and mouth cancers

        3.   spread to adjacent tissue and through bloodstream and lymphatic system

  B.   Sarcomas: found in muscle and bone and connective tissue found in the middle (mesodermal) layers of the body

        1.   spread through blood during early part of disease

  C.   Lymphomas: found in the lymphatic system

        1.   travels quickly throughout the body

        2.   e.g., Hodgkin's disease

  D.   Leukemia: found in blood-forming parts of the body including bone marrow and spleen

        1.   characterized by high white blood cell count

VI.   Types of cancer: categorized according to body part

  A.   Lung cancer

        1.   75 % of lung cancer related to smoking

        2.   rapid replacement of cells killed by smoke eventually produces a cancerous cell

        3.   smoker who quits for 10 years has a risk of lung cancer similar to a nonsmoker

        4.   symptoms: persistent cough, blood in the sputum, recurring bronchitis or pneumonia and chest pain

        5.   treatment: surgical removal of tumors, chemotherapy, radiation therapy

        6.   only 13% survive more than 5 years after diagnosis

  B.   Breast cancer

        1.   over past 60 years breast cancer has slowly and steadily increased

        2.   both men and women can develop it although more common in women

        3.   symptoms: lump, thickening, swelling, dimpling, skin irritation, distortion, nipple discharge, pain or tenderness of the breast

        4.   risk factors: age (over 50), family history especially in sister, mother or grandmother, sedentary lifestyle, never having children, not breast feeding, and having a first child after age 30.

        5.   some studies show a 30 % greater risk of breast cancer among women who drink 3 alcoholic drinks a week as compared to those who seldom or never drink

        6.   the more estrogen in a woman's body over her lifetime, the greater her risk of breast cancer (early menarche, late menopause and obesity increase estrogen)

        7.   studies of hormone treatment (hormone replacement therapy) find NO link to breast cancer

        8.   early detection is the best defense against breast cancer

            a.   women 20–40 years old, monthly breast self-exam, professional exam every 3 years

            b.   women 40–49 years old, monthly breast self-exam, professional exam yearly, baseline mammogram between ages 35 and 49

            c.   women over 50 years old, monthly breast self-exam, mammogram and clinical breast exam yearly: research evidence that this will cut breast cancer mortality in this age group by one third

        9.   treatments: lumpectomy, radical mastectomy, chemotherapy, and radiation therapy

        10.   five-year breast cancer survival rate has increased from 78 % in 1940 to 92% today

  C.   Skin cancer

        1.   if caught early, usually not life threatening

2.   3–5 % of skin cancers are malignant melanomas which spread quickly and are more dangerous

3.   risk factors: red or blond hair, freckling on the upper back, family history of melanomas, 3 or more severe sunburns as a teenager, 2–3 years outdoor work in the summer

4.   symptoms: change in a wart, mole or sore

5.   prevention:

   a.   avoiding excessive exposure to the sun or other artificial sources of ultraviolet light (indoor sunlamps/tanning lights)

   b.   wearing sunblock with a Sun Protection Factor (SPF) of at least 15

   c.   wearing a hat and long-sleeved shirt and long pants if possible

D.   Colon and rectal cancer

1.   third most common cancer for both men and women

2.   affects 156,000 yearly; 55,000 died in 1992

3.   men develop it more often than women

4.   adults over 50 years of age are at greatest risk

5.   risk factors: mostly lifestyle

   a.   diet high in fat and low in fiber

   b.   sedentary

6.   serious symptoms: blood in the stool, bleeding from the rectum, changes in bowel habits

7.   tend to spread slowly, which greatly increases survival following surgery

8.   prevention: annual digital rectal examination

E.   Prostate cancer

1.   second most deadly cancer for men, killing 32,000 men a year

2.   1:11 will suffer from it

3.   risk factors: greater than 45 years old, family history, a high-fat diet, multiple sexual partners, and a history of STDs

4.   African Americans are more susceptible to this cancer than males of other races; recommend they start screenings at age 45

5.   symptoms: vague and nonspecific, pain or difficulty when urinating, pain in the lower back or pelvis, and blood in the urine

6.   survival rate for those with localized cancer is 88 %

7.   prevention: digital rectal exams and prostate-specific antigen tests yearly after age 50

F.   Cervical and uterine cancer

   a.   yearly Pap test (more effective detecting cervical than uterine cancer)

   b.   risk factors: early age of first intercourse, multiple sex partners, cigarette smoking, and exposure to STDs

G.   Testicular cancer

1.   one of the few cancers to affect men between ages 15 and 34

2.   prevention: testicular self-examination

3.   symptoms: lumps or nodules on either testicle

VII.   Cancer prevention through diet

A.   Dietary guidelines to reduce cancer risk from the American Cancer Society

1.   maintain a desirable weight

2.   eat a varied diet

3.   include a variety of vegetables and fruits in your daily diet

4.   include cruciferous vegetables in your diet

5.   eat more high-fiber foods such as whole-wheat cereals, bread and pasta

6.   reduce total fat intake

7.   limit animal foods charred by grilling or broiling

8.   if you drink alcohol, do so in moderation

B.   Being 40 % overweight increases risk of colon, breast, gallbladder, prostate, ovarian and uterine cancers.

C.   Colorectal, stomach, breast, esophageal, and uterine cancers are linked to high-fat diets.

D.   Dietary fiber may help prevent colon cancer by retaining water which helps move fecal matter through the intestine more quickly; this shortens the time of exposure of the large intestine wall to any cancer-causing agents that might be in the fecal matter.

E.   Adding antioxidants to the diet may prevent gene damage inflicted by free radicals which may be a direct cause of cancer (see nutrition in chapter 6, vitamins A, C, and E).

F.   Heavy use of alcohol is associated with an increased risk of mouth, larynx, throat, esophageal, and liver cancers.

VIII.   Cancer prevention through exercise

A.   Regular, moderate to vigorous physical activity reduces the risk of several cancers, especially colon cancer.

1.   sedentary individuals have 30–100 % more risk of colon cancer than those who are active

2.   exercise stimulates intestinal walls, encouraging fecal matter movement, which decreases time for carcinogens to be in contact with the intestinal walls

3.   may also be that active people are more apt to eat a high-fiber, low-fat diet

B.   Poorly fit individuals are at higher risk for death from cancer than those with average or good fitness.

1.   for men, poor fitness is associated with 3–5 times more risk

2.   for women, good fitness reduces risk to 1/16th that of unfit women

C.   Women who are physically active during their reproductive lifetime (teens to age 40) have less incidence of breast and reproductive organ cancers.

1.   one study from the Southern California Norris Cancer Center reported that:

a.   1–3 hours of exercise a week can bring a 20–30 % reduction in risk of breast cancer; 4 or more hours per week can bring a 60% reduction of risk

b.   women who were athletes in college had fewer cases of breast and reproductive cancer probably because of later menarche and earlier menopause, which reduces exposure to estrogen over a lifetime

c.   you do not have to be an athlete to get protective benefits from exercise; moderate to vigorous aerobic exercise will provide comparable levels of protection

IX.   Detecting cancer

A.   The earlier cancer is detected, the better the chances of survival.

B.   Cancer can be diagnosed using special computers and high-tech imaging machines.

1.   magnetic resonance imagery (MRI)

2.   computer axial tomography (a CAT scan)

C.   Cancer can be diagnosed by analyzing a sample of suspected cancer tissue (biopsy) removed from the body using a small needle.

X. Treating cancer
  A. Surgery
    1. works on localized cancers
    2. often used in conjunction with radiation therapy (destroys any remaining cancer cells)
  B. Radiation therapy
    1. used with surgery
    2. used to treat cancers that are difficult to remove surgically or that have not responded well to drug or immune treatments
  C. Chemotherapy
    1. uses powerful drugs or hormones to kill spreading cancer cells
  D. Immunotherapy
    1. method which stimulates the body's own immune system to attack spreading cancer cells
    2. patient is injected with antibodies or vaccines grown from the patient's own tumor cells

XI. Living with cancer
  A. A cancer diagnosis is no longer a death sentence; the survival rates continue to improve, especially with early diagnosis.
  B. Workshops, support groups, and computer support groups are available.
  C. Today there are at least 8 million cancer survivors in the United States.

XII. Diabetes
  A. Diabetes mellitus is a common metabolic disease that occurs either because the pancreas fails to produce sufficient insulin or because the insulin being produced is not used efficiently.
    1. insulin is a hormone that makes blood glucose available to cells
    2. insufficient insulin results in an accumulation of glucose (sugar) in the blood
    3. kidneys can't process all the glucose so it spills over into the urine and is excreted
  B. Diabetes is the 7th leading cause of death.
    1. 30,000 die annually from it
    2. 300,000 die from complications stemming from it
    3. estimated 10 million Americans have it; 4 million of which are unaware they have it
    4. those with diabetes have twice the risk of heart disease and stroke
  C. Diabetes is the number one cause of blindness in the U.S.
  D. Diabetes accounts for one-third of all cases of kidney failure.
  E. There are two types of diabetes: Type I and Type II.
    1. Type I Diabetes
      a. insulin-dependent because the cells in the pancreas that normally produces it are destroyed by the body's own immune system
      b. usually strikes suddenly in childhood, can be anytime before age 35
      c. believed to be linked to a viral infection
      d. treatment: insulin replacement therapy through daily insulin injections
    2. Type II diabetes
      a. occurrence is gradual usually striking overweight adults over age 35
      b. non-insulin dependent
      c. 90% of cases of diabetes are type II
      d. risk factors: family history, being overweight, being sedentary, race

(1) Native Americans, African American, and Hispanics have a higher risk than Caucasians

    e. treatment: maintain regular blood glucose levels through regular exercise, normal body weight, and consistent dietary intervention

(1) American Diabetes Association recommends type II diabetics consume 60 % of their calories from complex carbohydrates and reduce consumption of sugar by avoiding them or using sugar substitutes

  F. Exercise and diabetes

    a. diabetics may participate in (and are encouraged to do) many forms of exercise

    b. the amount and intensity of exercise should be determined in consultation with a physician

    c. exercise increases blood flow, which in some cases mobilizes too much injected insulin

(1) hypoglycemia or low blood sugar can occur if high concentrations of insulin build up and sweep glucose out of the blood

(2) to prevent hypoglycemia, the timing and placement of insulin injections should be set in consultation with a physician

(3) diabetics should carry a sugar-type snack to eat in case of low blood sugar, as inadequate circulation of blood sugar to the brain can result in unconsciousness, even death

XIII. Headaches

  A. Common noninfectious condition caused by stress or by physiological changes in the body

  B. Twenty percent of Americans experience severe headaches with so much pain as to cause dizziness, nausea, and even temporary visual impairment

  C. There are four types of headaches: tension, psychological, secondary, and migraine.

    1. tension headaches: caused by involuntary muscle tension

      a. may be the result of stress, boredom, fatigue, physical labor, or poor posture

      b. treatment: mild pain relievers, relaxation and stress reduction

      c. treatment for chronic tension headaches: eliminate the cause

    2. psychological headaches: caused by anxiety, depression, mental and emotional stress

      a. treatment: social and psychological therapies designed to relieve depression and stress

    3. secondary headaches: a side effect of some other underlying condition

      a. causes: flu, fasting, hypertension, excessive heat, allergies, bodily pain or injury, poor eyesight

      b. treatment: eliminate the underlying cause, mild pain relievers for pain

    4. migraine headaches: caused by rapid constriction and dilation of blood vessels in the brain—no known reason for this phenomenon

      a. accompanied by a release of chemicals that inflame some of the brain tissue

      b. severe pain lasts minutes or days, usually on one side of the head

      c. may suffer temporary visual impairment and hypersensitivity to sun

      d. treatments: pain killers only mildly effective, consult with physician for new treatments

XIV. Allergies

A. The allergic response is the result of an over reaction of a person's own immune system in an attempt to eliminate allergens (allergy-causing substances).
   1. histamines dilate blood vessels and increase mucus membranes; too much histamine results in congestion, runny nose, watery eyes
B. Common allergens are: pollen, mold, animal dander, synthetic materials, and dust.
C. An allergic reaction may also be triggered by foods, drugs, and insect bites.
D. Symptoms: running nose, watery eyes, sneezing, nasal congestion, itching of the ears, nose and throat, and occasionally hives.
E. Anaphylactic shock is a rare allergic response that drops blood pressure drastically, restricts respiration severely, and if not treated in time, results in death.
F. Allergies tend to be inherited.
G. People in rural settings are exposed to more allergens and tend to have higher allergy rates than those in urban settings.
H. Detection: health history, detailed list of symptoms, allergy skin test.
I. Treatment: avoidance of irritating substance, desensitizing the immune system with a series of shots containing minute amounts of allergens.

XV. Asthma
A. A chronic disease of the lung airways characterized by spasm of the muscles surrounding the airway and inflammation of the airway.
B. Causes are allergens, exercise, smoking, cold air, pollutants, stress or infection
C. Treatments are prescription inhalers which spray a small dose of muscle relaxant, brochodilator, or anti-inflammatory medications into the lungs.
D. Cases of asthma on the rise, increased by a third in the last 10 years, deaths due to asthma doubled, reason unknown
E. Most severely affected by asthma are adults over 65, children, and African Americans living in inner-city communities.
F. Exercise-induced asthma (EIA) is also on the rise.
G. EIA can be effectively managed
   1. seventy 1984 Olympic athletes had EIA, 40 medaled
   2. treatment: inhale a dose of prescribed medication 15–30 minutes prior to exercise and any time during exercise that symptoms appear (see also chapter 2)

BEHAVIOR BOOSTS: STAGE-BASED STUDENT ACTIVITIES

Precontemplator
- If you go outside today, watch for people working on tans; they're precontemplators.
- Remember that if you tan now, you may pay later.
- Watch a public service announcement made by a lung cancer victim.
- Think about the fact that the risk of some cancers may be lessened by the lifestyle choices we make.

Contemplator
- Can you think of someone who has cancer? How has the diagnosis affected his or her life?
- Memorize the cancer warning signs.
- Think about how much money you could save if you didn't go to a tanning salon. You could buy some new clothes or save the money instead.

Preparer
- Eat a fruit or vegetable for lunch today.
- Take a few minutes to closely inspect your skin for possible skin cancers.
- Avoid or reduce your consumption of high-fat foods today.

Action Taker
- Choose to eat broccoli, cauliflower, or cabbage for dinner tonight.
- Start the practice of monthly breast or testicular self-examinations by doing yours tonight.
- Think about the positive changes you have made in your life since you began practicing cancer prevention.

Maintainer
- Do you remember the seven cancer warning signs? If you don't, you should review them and commit them to memory.
- Review Chapter 6 to find ways to jazz up your low-fat diet.
- If your exercise routine is getting boring, maybe it's time for a change. If you usually exercise alone, get a friend to join you or sign up for an aerobic class with other motivated people who will keep you company.

ADDITIONAL STUDENT ACTIVITIES

Activity 1: Self-examinations for Early Detection of Cancer

Follow the directions for a breast self-examination on page 239.
Follow the directions for a testicular self-examination on page 240.

Activity 2: Assessment Checklist for Cancer Risk

This assessment checklist is found in this manual at the end of this chapter.

LABS

Lab 10.1 What Can I Do? (pages 249–250)

RESOURCES

Suggested Reading

Blum, A., ed. *The cigarette underworld—A front line report on the war against your lungs.* New York: Lyle Stuart. 1985.

Fiore, N.A. *The road back to health: Coping with the emotional side of cancer.* New York: Bantam Books, 1985.

Prescott, D.M., and A.S. Flexer. *Cancer—The misguided cell*, 3rd ed. New York: Charles Scribner's Sons, 1986.

Organizations

American Academy of Allergy, Asthma, &
Immunology
611 East Wells Street
Milwaukee, WI 53202
Tel (414) 272-6071
Web site: http://www.AAAAI.org

American Cancer Society
Web site:
http://www2.acan.net~amcancer/cancer.org

American Council for Headache Education
19 Mantua Road
Mt Royal, NJ 08061
Tel: (609) 423-0258
Fax: (609) 423-0082
Web site: www.achenet.org

American Diabetes Association
1660 Duke Street
Alexandria, VA 22314
Tel: see web site for local phone numbers
Web site: http://www.diabetes.org

Association of Community Cancer Centers
11600 Nebel Street, Suite 201
Rockville, MD 20852

Cancer Connection
Web site: http://www.cancer-connection.com

Health Promotion Service Branch
Division of Resources, Centers and Community
Activities
National Cancer Institute
Department of Health and Human Services
Building 31, Room 10A-18
9000 Rockville Pike
Bethesda, MD 20205
(800) 4-CANCER

Additional Local and Community Resources

Blue Cross/Blue Shield
Cancer Information Service(CIS)
State and County Health Departments
American Lung Association

ASSESSMENT CHECKLIST FOR CANCER RISK

For each question, select the response that best describes you; record the point value in the space provided. Total your points for each section separately.

1. Sex   ____
   - 2   Male
   - 1   Female

2. Age   ____
   - 1   39 or less
   - 2   40–49
   - 5   50–59
   - 7   60 and over

3. Smoking   ____
   - 8   smoker
   - 1   nonsmoker

4. Type of smoking   ____
   - 10   Current smoker of cigarettes or little cigars
   - 3   Pipe and/or cigar, but not cigarettes
   - 2   Ex-cigarette smoker
   - 1   Nonsmoker

5. Amount of cigarettes smoked per day   ____
   - 1   zero (0)
   - 5   Less than ½ pack
   - 9   ½ to 1 pack
   - 15   1 to 2 packs
   - 20   2 or more packs

6. Type of cigarette[a]   ____
   - 10   High tar/nicotine
   - 9   Medium tar/nicotine
   - 7   Low tar/nicotine
   - 1   Nonsmoker

Source: American Cancer Society
[a]Tar/nicotine levels:
High: 20 + mg. tar/1.3 – mg. nicotine; Medium: 16–19 mg. tar/1.1–1.2 mg. nicotine; Low: 15 mg. or less tar/1.0 mg. or less nicotine

7. Duration of smoking   ____
   - 1   Never smoked
   - 3   Ex-smoker
   - 5   Up to 15 years
   - 10   15–25 years
   - 20   25 or more years

8. Type of industrial work   ____
   - 3   Mining
   - 7   Asbestos
   - 5   Uranium and radioactive products

Lung total   ____

Colon and Rectal Cancer

1. Age   ____
   - 10   39 or less
   - 20   40–59
   - 50   60 and over

2. Has anyone in your immediate family ever had: ____
   - 20   Colon cancer
   - 10   One or more colon polyps
   - 1   Neither

3. Have you ever had: ____
   - 100   Colon cancer
   - 40   One or more colon polyps
   - 20   Ulcerative colitis
   - 10   Cancer of the breast or uterus
   - 1   None

4. Bleeding from the rectum (other than obvious hemorrhoids or piles)   ____
   - 75   Yes
   - 1   No

Colon and rectal total   ____

Skin Cancer

1. Frequent work or play in the sun   ____
   10 Yes
   1 No

2. Work in mines, around coal tars, or   ____
   around radioactivity
   10 Yes
   1 No

3. Complexion-fair skin and/or light skin   ____
   10 Yes
   1 No

Skin total   ____

Breast Cancer (Women Only)

1. Age group   ____
   10 20–34
   40 35–49
   90 50 and over

2. Racial group   ____
   5 Asian
   20 African American
   25 Non-Hispanic White
   10 Hispanic

3. Family history   ____
   30 Mother, sister, aunt, or
      grandmother with breast cancer
   10 None

4. Your history   ____
   25 Previous lumps or cysts
   10 No breast disease
   100 Previous breast cancer

5. Maternity   ____
   10 1st pregnancy before 25
   15 1st pregnancy after 25
   20 No pregnancies

Breast cancer total   ____

Cervical Cancer (Women Only)

1. Age group   ____
   10 Less than 25
   20 25–39
   30 40–54
   30 55 and over

2. Racial group   ____
   10 Asian
   20 African American
   10 Non-Hispanic White
   20 Hispanic

3. Number of pregnancies   ____
   10 0
   20 1 to 3
   30 4 and over

4. Viral infections   ____
   10 Herpes and other viral infections
      or ulcer formations on the vagina
   1 Never

5. Age at first intercourse   ____
   40 Before 15
   30 15–19
   20 20–24
   10 25 and over
   5 Never

6. Bleeding between periods or after   ____
   intercourse
   40 Yes
   1 no

Cervical total   ____

(See analysis on the next page.)

Analysis

If your *lung* total is:

24 or less	You have a low risk for lung cancer.
25–49	You may be a light smoker and would benefit from quitting.
50–74	As a moderate smoker, your risks for lung and upper respiratory tract cancer are increased. If you stop smoking now, these risks will decrease.
75 or over	As a heavy cigarette smoker, your risks for lung and upper respiratory tract cancer are greatly increased. You should stop smoking now. See your physician if you have possible signs of lung cancer (nagging cough, hoarseness, persistent sore in the mouth or throat).

If your *colon and rectal* total is:

29 or less	You are at low risk for colon and rectal cancer.
30–69	You are at moderate risk. Testing by your physician may be indicated.
70 or over	You are at high risk. You should see your physician for the following tests: digital rectal exam, stool occult blood test, and (where applicable) proctoscopic exam.

Numerical risks for *skin* cancer are difficult to state. For instance, a person with a dark complexion can work longer in the sun and be less likely to develop cancer than a light-complected person. Furthermore, a person wearing a long sleeved shirt and wide-brimmed hat may work in the sun and be less at risk than a person who wears a bathing suit only a short period. The risk goes up greatly with age. If you answered "yes" to any question, you need to protect your skin from the sun or any other toxic material. Changes in moles, warts, or skin sores are very important and need to be seen by your physician.

If your *breast* total is:

100 or less	You are at low risk. You should practice monthly BSE and have your breasts examined by a physician as part of a cancer-related check-up.
101–199	You are at moderate risk. You should practice monthly BSE and have your breasts examined by a physician as part of a cancer-related checkup. Periodic mammograms should be included as directed by your physician.
200 or over	You are at high risk. You should practice monthly BSE and have professional examinations more often. See your physician for the examinations recommended for you.

If your *cervical* total is:

40–69	You are at low risk. Your physician will advise you about how often you should have a Pap test.
70–99	You are at moderate risk. More frequent Pap tests may be required.
100 or more	You are at high risk. You should have a Pap test and pelvic exam as advised by your physician.

Understanding and Managing Stress

Chapter 11

CHAPTER SUMMARY

Stress is a multifaceted phenomenon. It has been studied from psychological, biological, and social perspectives, all of which provide us with part of the "picture" of stress. Stress-management techniques vary according to the nature of the stress.

There are many kinds of stressors, both good (eustress) and bad stress (distress). Stressors can be beyond our control or preventable. Often the stressor does not itself cause stress; rather, our perception of the stressor is the problem. The intensity and duration of distress, the resources available, and our coping abilities all determine the impact of the stress. Being aware of how our perception can shape events and affect others can also help to reduce or prevent stressful situations.

Sources of stress vary a great deal from person to person, as do personality, hardiness, and perception. An effective stress program must be tailored to the individual, and as with any behavior change program, both short- and long-term goals should be established. When stress, anxiety, and depression are too high, professional help is needed. On the other hand, sometimes just a little help is needed to get through a tough period and friends, families, and community resources can make a difference.

Challenge is good for personal and professional growth. The important thing is to prevent challenge from becoming chronic distress. Letting off steam through exercise, eating right, getting plenty of sleep, and maintaining a sense of humor can all help you keep a healthy perspective.

LEARNING OBJECTIVES

The student will be able to:

- define and give examples of positive and negative stress.
- understand the multifaceted nature of stress and define it accordingly.
- explain the basic tenets of biological (physiological), psychological, and social stress theory.
- list the personality traits most associated with a stressful lifestyle and those of "hardy" individuals.
- explain how arousal, performance, and stress are related.
- recognize symptoms of, and responses to, stress in oneself and others.
- select and practice one or more coping and stress reduction strategies.

PERSONAL PROFILE

Arsenio Hall

Have you ever been under so much stress that you feel overwhelmed? This is a common feeling for individuals who carry large work loads or who are constantly faced with deadlines. As the host and executive producer of the "Arsenio Hall Show," Arsenio Hall understands what it feels like to be overwhelmed. The constant push to do better and accomplish more has caused some of Arsenio's best friends to say to him, "You're gonna kill yourself. You need outlets." For Arsenio, stress reduction is a major element of success.

So how does this popular entertainer and businessman reduce the stress in his life? Arsenio's solution to stress is painting! "I love what it does as far as stress and relaxation," he says with excitement. "All of a sudden, I found myself at my house, with the phone off, in a room, for hours. And every time I looked at a painting, I could almost see how I was feeling that period, what I was going through."

Most of the paintings he completes remain in his home. Occasionally, he gives one to a close friend or relative, and the members of his staff are able to enjoy one that hangs on the wall of his Paramount lot studio. It's an abstract acrylic done in hurried strokes of blue, and he's not likely to explain what it means. For him, the meaning of the work is not as important as the reason for the work. Arsenio understands the need to have a balance in his profession; he has learned that too much work can lead to too much stress. Without the stress relief he gets from painting, his closest friends can attest that Arsenio would literally work himself to death.

Harris, Joanne. Arsenio Hall. Comedy is his sword, painting is his shield. *American Visions*, Feb/Mar, 14-17, 1994.

CONTENT OUTLINE

I.   Life requires stress.
    A.   The right amount of stress stimulates the mind and body and keeps us healthy.
    B.   Too much stress is bad—distress.
        1.   75–90% of all doctor's visits are related to stress
        2.   burn out is a common form of stress, can be work-related
    C.   Too little stress is bad–hypostress.
        1.   boredom, loneliness, apathy may result from too few challenges, etc.

II.   Stress can be defined and studied from several perspectives.
    A.   Stress is something external to the person that causes mental and/or physical tension and arousal.
        1.   the term "stressor" is frequently used in place of stress in this definition
            a.   stressors can be physical, emotional or social
    B.   Stress is the internal state of a person.
        1.   the term "strain" is sometimes used in place of stress in this definition
            a.   strain refers to both the physiological and emotional states of a person
                (1)   when a demand is placed on the body, the body reacts by rising to a higher level of arousal
                    (a)   to defend itself against something harmful or to perform at a level needed to meet the challenge

        (2)   emotional responses, such as anger and joy also constitute your internal state

C.   Stress is what arises from a transaction between a person and the environment.

    a.   stress is a combination of the stressor and the way the stressor is perceived or interpreted by the individual

        (1)   if a person believes that a situation will result in loss, harm, threat, or challenge, the individual will experience stress

            (a)   the environmental condition does not create stress by itself

            (b)   the situation and the person's appraisal of the situation work together to create the stress

III.   Stress and physical wellness

    A.   Physical stress like exercise strengthens the body.

    B.   Too much physical stress can lead to weakness, injury, and overuse syndromes like carpal tunnel and tendonitis.

    C.   Human beings are social creatures by nature.

        1.   lack of social interaction can be as harmful (lack of social stress or stimulation)

            a.   babies whose basic physical needs are met but who are left alone rather than cuddled and caressed show poorer weight gains and delayed neurological development

            b.   recent studies have found that a mother's caresses seem to help moderate production of a hormone that affects the body's reaction to stress

            c.   lack of social interaction in children and adults can manifest itself as loneliness, isolation, and doubts of self-worth

        2.   too much emotional and social stress can have a negative impact on health

            a.   abusive, degrading, or highly demanding relationships can create excessive interpersonal tension

            b.   common social and emotional stressors include employment conditions, financial status, racial acceptance, balancing the obligations of home and work responsibilities

        3.   social and emotional stress balances are achieved by developing positive relationships and having at least one other person you can depend on

            a.   married people live longer than unmarried individuals

            b.   women giving birth with someone there to emotionally support them have fewer complications

IV.   Stress and spiritual wellness

    A.   Spiritual stress may include ethical and moral decision making, feelings of guilt, and the acceptance or rejection of religious beliefs.

        1.   too little spiritual stress may result in a failure to resolve issues such as death and the meaning of one's life

        2.   too much spiritual stress can manifest itself in spiritual coercion (such as cults), or in the kind of overwhelming guilt that results in suicide

        3.   finding a spiritual balance provides comfort, joy, and a sense of purpose

V.   Stress and mental wellness

    A.   The human brain, our intellect, thrives on being stimulated and challenged.

        1.   a lack of stimulation can result in boredom, a loss of motivation, failure to progress and even regression

        2.   those who are intellectually stimulated and challenged tend to thrive

           a.   children who are encouraged to read at home tend to do better in school and their linguistic development may have long reaching health effects

              (1)   the Nuns Studies discovered that those nuns who demonstrated more complex linguistic patterns early in life were less likely to develop Alzheimer's disease

  B.   Too much mental stress is bad and may result in frustration and burnout.

           a.   mental challenges that exceed a person's capabilities and coping abilities cause distress

           b.   too much mental stress hinders development and interferes with motivation

           c.   stress arises from difficult situations where a person has too few resources and limited decision-making control

VI.   The stress continuum ranges from bad (distress) to good stress (eustress).

  A.   While eustress can cause the same physiological responses as distress, it is not linked to stress-related disease.

        1.   eustress is not chronic like distress can be and therefore the individual returns more quickly to homeostasis

  B.   Person does not have control over most stressors but does have control over how she or he perceives and reacts to a stressor.

        1.   one person's distress can be another person's eustress

        2.   both real and imagined stressors will result in a stress response

VII.   Stress and performance

  A.   Arousal is a form of stimulation (stress) that affects performance.

        1.   if you are excited you will perform better than if you are not particularly aroused

        2.   too much arousal can cause a decrease in performance quality

  B.   The inverted "U" hypothesis (Yerkes-Dodson Law) describes the relationship between arousal, stress, and performance.

        1.   low arousal and excessive arousal result in low performance

        2.   the top of the inverted "U" represents the amount of arousal that results in best performance

        3.   a greater amount of arousal is needed for what are referred to as "simple tasks" such as strength, speed, muscular endurance activities than for "complex tasks" such as accuracy, agility, and balancing activities

VIII. Theories about stress

  A.   Stress is so broad a subject that researchers and scholars have studied it from a variety of perspectives.

        1.   physiologists study the body's physical reaction to stress

           a.   e.g., elevated heart rate, increased hormone production and higher rates of illness

        2.   psychologists examine mental and emotional stress

           a.   issues such as perception and personality

        3.   human engineers and sociologists concentrate on how environmental conditions and societal pressures influence stress

           a.   e.g., war, work environments, crowding, noise, etc.

  B.   Stress and the physical response

        1.   Walter Cannon introduced the ideas of homeostasis and fight or flight.

a. defined homeostasis as the tendency of organisms to maintain a stable internal environment
    (1) initial or low level environmental stressor could be withstood and the organisms would adapt and bounce back, restoring homeostasis
    (2) high intensity or continued physical stressors could result in a disturbance of homeostasis that could ultimately lead to a breakdown of biological systems
b. described the physical response to a stressor in terms of a fight or flight reaction

2. Hans Selye's pioneer research established the formal study of stress.
    a. influenced by Walter Cannon
    b. defined stress as the nonspecific response of the body to any demand made upon it
        (1) cited common physiological responses which appear to occur regardless of the nature of the illness (e.g., elevated heart rate and body temperature) as evidence of the nonspecific response to stress
    c. named good stress "eustress" and bad stress "distress"
    d. concluded that the body reacts in a similar way to both distress and eustress
    e. called the body's physical responses to stress the "stress response"
        (1) describes the stress response as a three-stage syndrome (see general adaptation syndrome below)
        (2) during chronic stress, Selye argued, the body acts like a chain giving out at its weakest link
        (3) people can manifest different stress symptoms and diseases with chronic stress because their "weak link" can differ from someone else's
        (4) today researchers recognize that the stress response is not only physical but also psychological

3. General adaptation syndrome (G.A.S.): a three-stage stress response to explain how the body responds to sudden stress, chronic stress, and excessive stress, resulting in physical collapse
    a. the alarm stage
        (1) the immediate response to a stressor
            (a) the sympathetic branch of the autonomic nervous system responds by quickly eliciting body changes needed to either fight or run away (flight) from a perceived threat
            (b) senses sharpen, become more alert, epinephrine (adrenaline) pours into the bloodstream, heart rate increases, and muscles tense in readiness
    b. the resistance stage
        (1) in the case of a sudden, high-intensity stressor, the alarm response occurs and then dissipates, followed by a resistance phase in which the adaptive energy remains elevated
        (2) when stress becomes chronic, the body begins to view it as a normal condition and adjusts to establish a new level of homeostasis

(3) continued stress leads to exhaustion; if allowed to continue, chronically fatiguing stress may diminish the body's ability to resist illness

c. the exhaustion stage

(1) occurs when stress is very intense or lasts too long

(a) when the body can no longer resist, it slumps into exhaustion characterized by an inability to work, physical collapse, and potentially death

(b) this type of exhaustion can occur even when a person is eating a nutritious diet and getting enough sleep

i) according to Selye, a person's adaptive energy reserve, a stockpile of energy available for adapting to difficult situations, can become depleted; regular energy levels will return to normal with rest but the adaptive energy reserve cannot be replenished

ii) scientists today do not necessarily agrees with Selye's theory; he explains the physiological phenomenon of stress but does not address psychosocial issues, cognitive processes or the selection, use and effectiveness of coping strategies

C. Psychological aspects of stress

1. different positions have been taken by physiological and psychological theorists regarding stress

a. J. W. Mason challenged Selye's biologically based theory by showing that the physiological system is sensitive to, and influenced by, emotional input

b. Lazarus argues that the nature and severity of a stress disorder is tied to the interaction between environmental demands and the quality of the individual's emotional response and the coping process selected.

(1) one of the most prominent psychological theories of stress is the cognitive transactional model of stress by Lazarus

(a) stress is described as a relationship between demands and the power to deal with them without suffering unreasonable and destructive costs

i) demands are determined by an individual's perception rather than by an absolute value

a) this means that demands may be considered very high by one person and low by another

b) the same person may even perceive the demands as different at different times

(2) chronic stress may have cognitive side effects such as emotional outbursts, anger displacement, distorted perception, and the lessening ability to plan rationally and make decisions

D. Perception and stress

1. the way people interpret and frame things can create stress, not only for themselves but for others

          a.   perceptual differences can easily lead to miscommunication, one of the greatest sources of interpersonal tension

             (1)   miscommunication often occurs when people work from different frames of reference

                (a)   gender differences in communication can cause tension

                (b)   cultural backgrounds can create funny or disastrous mishaps

2.   the actual stressor does not dictate a response; the perception of the demand of the stressor and the ability to meet the demand determine the response

3.   cognitive interventions can be applied when problems of perceptual origin are identified

E.   Personality and stress

1.   Four major types of personalities have been recognized.

          a.   Type A, hard driving, ambitious, competitive, high-strung, and high achieving

             (1)   control is a major factor in managing stress and Type A people are often in a position to control important job and lifestyle decisions, which may help them control their stress levels

             (2)   hostility and anger can lead to heart disease

          b.   Type B, relaxed and easygoing

             (1)   can experience stress if they are passive-aggressive

          c.   Type C, a blend of Type A and B without the aggressive hostility that a Type A can exhibit; is the most stress-resistant type

          d.   Type E, are the "please everyone" type

             (1)   may suffer from the feeling that they have not accomplished enough or that their efforts are inadequate

             (2)   experience guilt for not doing something or including someone; stress runs high for this group

2.   Suzanne Kobasa has studied stress and personality and identified characteristics of what she calls "hardy" personalities.

          a.   hardy people suffer fewer stress-related problems

          b.   hardy people look upon change as a natural occurrence and accept new developments as exciting challenges

3.   difficult to change a personality but awareness of personality type helps people avoid stressful situations

4.   there is some genetic-based research that suggests some people may be more predisposed for stress-related illness

F.   Social aspects of stress

1.   social stress theorists study how stress results from the relationship between individual and society

          a.   stress may be the result of a conflict between desire for something and the inability to obtain it

2.   life change theory explains stress in terms of the changes in our lives that require adaptive energy

          a.   daily hassles and small irritating problems may be more significant to health risk than major stressors

3.   environmental-ecological theory, considered a social theory, examines the stress caused by our surroundings (e.g., loud noises, crowding, poor air quality, bright or dim lighting, and chemical hazards)

G.   The interdisciplinary approach to stress management

    1.   psychoneuroimmunology suggests that psychological issues, including stress, can influence the health of the immune system and vice versa

    2.   biopsychosocial model for health and illness encourages the physician to consider not only the biological aspects of illness but also the psychological and social aspects

IX.   Techniques for managing stress

A.   The stress survival kit

    1.   identify the stressors in your life (look for symptoms and trace back to cause)

    2.   take control (preplan when possible)

    3.   accept your limitations (set priorities. let go of things you can't change)

    4.   change your attitude towards stressors you can't change

    5.   use stress-management strategies to reduce or escape distress

B.   Applying cognitive interventions

    1.   if thoughts and emotions can influence the stress response, then "thinking" interventions ought to be able to alleviate distress

        a.   you must first recognize how you are "thinking" yourself into distress

        b.   change thinking from a negative to a more positive outlook

    2.   forms of cognitive interventions include reframing, positive self-talk, and imagery

C.   Applying physiological interventions

    1.   techniques that relax the body help relax the mind

    2.   relaxing the body relieves muscle tension

    3.   forms of relaxation include progressive relaxation, autogenic training, meditation, and biofeedback

D.   Other stress management techniques include asking for help, creative problem solving, effective communication. and time management.

X.   A closer look at stress interventions

A.   Reframing

    1.   people tend to filter other people's actions through their own frame of reference and then pass judgment—instead, look for clues and try to put yourself in the other person's shoes

    2.   have a choice whether to view a situation from a good or bad perspective

    3.   seeing the glass as "half full" is less stressful

    4.   rationalizing is different from reframing because the truth of a situation can be lost during rationalizing

B.   Positive Self-talk

    1.   listen to your inner voice; a journal is a good way to do this

    2.   replace negative statements with positive ones

    3.   consider self-esteem exercises/workshops

C.   Imagery

    1.   involves the use of visualization to imagine yourself in. and successfully handling, stressful situations

    2.   imagination is a powerful tool

    3.   opportunity to work through scenarios in your head before trying them

D. Asking for help
 1. recognizing the need for and accepting help shows a strength of character
 2. a social support network has been shown to lower stress
 3. learning to be assertive can help during times when you feel unsure of yourself and can assist in overcoming feeling of unworthiness

E. Solving problems creatively
 1. brainstorm with your friend and see whether you can come up with creative solutions
 2. win-win solutions lower stress for all involved

F. Working on communication skills
 1. being an effective communicator prevents misunderstandings and facilitates interaction

G. Managing time
 1. a shortage of time is one of the chief complaints of people and a major source of stress
 2. develop time-management skills
  a. prioritize
  b. make a daily plan
  c. keep a journal to find out where time goes
  d. set aside personal work time
  e. handle paper once—make a decision the first time
  f. break big projects into manageable pieces
  g. limit interruptions when possible
  h. do the most difficult projects first
  i. delegate
  j. don't obsess over perfectionism
  k. learn to say no

H. Learn to relax
 1. when arousal is too high, performance declines
 2. when performance declines, people get frustrated and their anxiety creates more tension, which in turn makes performance even worse
 3. relaxation techniques break this vicious cycle
 4. techniques require several months to fully achieve but benefits will be acquired sooner

I. Progressive relaxation
 1. a technique developed by Edmond Jacobson that systematically relaxes your skeletal muscles, which will also have the effect of relaxing nearby organs and involuntary muscles
  a. alternately tensing and relaxing muscles in a predetermined order

J. Autogenic training
 1. is a series of six psycho-physiologic exercises developed by Johannes H. Schultz
 2. uses mental images of things like warmth and heaviness to induce relaxation

K. Meditation
 1 is a form of deep relaxation and concentration that allows you to free yourself from the bombardment of conscious thought and achieve a more objective perspective
 2 transcendental meditation uses breathing and visualization and muscular relaxation techniques

L.   Biofeedback

    3   teaches you how to exert voluntary control over certain functions of the autonomic nervous system; this control can then be used to relieve tension

    4   physicians use a number of common instruments to monitor physiological responses, including EKG, or pulse monitor for heart rate. EEG for brain waves, and computer-generated visual representation of respiration rate and blood pressure

M.   Laughter

    5   it is impossible to laugh and stay tense for very long

    6   laughter diffuses physical tension and triggers a relaxation response

XI   Seeking a balanced level of stress

A.   People who suffer from too little stress or hypostress can be bored, lonely and isolated. This can be combated by seeking out stimulation.

B.   People who are over stressed, frustrated, burned out, etc., can use stress interventions to diffuse and eliminate stress.

C.   Taking care of yourself helps balance stress.

    7   eat right

    8   get enough sleep

    9   exercise

    10   limit or avoid alcohol and caffeine

    11   avoid tobacco and drugs

    12   seek out challenges

    13   look at life from a positive frame of reference

    14   limit what you take on and get help when you need it

BEHAVIOR BOOSTS: STAGE-BASED STUDENT ACTIVITIES

Precontemplator
- Ask family members or close friends whether they think you are overly stressed (hyperstressed). Ask them to give you examples of how the stress negatively affects you or those around you.
- Take notice of the times when you feel "stressed out" and experience symptoms like headaches, anger, hassles, lack of time, etc.
- Think back over your medical appointments to see if you have seen a physician for anything that might be stress-related. If you are in counseling, talk with your counselor about how you are handling the stress in your life.
- Talk to people you admire for their even temperament and organized lifestyle. Ask them how they do it.
- Take a stress test and reflect on the results.

Contemplator
- Think about the advantages of better managing your stress.
- Think about the consequences of your stress level. Besides affecting you, whom does it affect?
- Consider how other people's behaviors affect your stress level or ability to cope.
- Look at the action taker behavior boosts and see if there are any actions you would consider taking.
- Find out where you can get information on stress management. For example, check for courses at the American Red Cross, on campus, or through your employer.
- Talk to people who are handling stressful situations well and ask them how they do it.

Preparer

- Identify the top stressor in your life and learn about how you can minimize the effects of this stressor. Or identify a challenge or stimulating activity you would like to add to your life.
- Write a behavior change goal and set a start date.
- Enroll in a course in stress or time management, medication, or exercise.
- Make an appointment with a knowledgeable person, such as a professor, counselor, physician, or spiritual leader to learn more about stress management.
- Get a medical checkup to rule out medical reasons for possible stress-related symptoms such as headaches and fatigue.
- Practice saying no to unwanted commitments through role playing.
- Rehearse what you want to say to someone with whom you have a conflict that is resulting in stress, and then make an appointment to talk with him or her.
- Look at the action taker list and experiment with some of the ideas listed there in an effort to find something that works for you and fits in with your lifestyle.

Action Taker

- Get a massage.
- Go for a walk or a run, or turn on the music and dance around the room.
- Pet a friendly animal
- Stretch or perform yoga, or take a class in one of the martial arts.
- Prioritize.
- Delegate.
- Take a warm bath or shower.
- Tell a joke, read, or watch something funny.
- Hit a punching bag instead of a person or valued item.
- Take a deep breath and exhale slowly.
- Tense your shoulders (shoulder shrug) and then relax.
- Place a picture of someone or something you like nearby and look at it. For example, it could be a vacation place you'll be traveling to soon.
- Play an upbeat tune and take a mini-break for three to five minutes.
- Use humor or politeness to diffuse someone else's stress. Diffusing theirs will reduce yours.
- Use a relaxation strategy such as meditation, exercise, progressive relaxation, autogenic training, or biofeedback.
- Use a cognitive stress management strategy, such as reframing or positive self-talk.
- To identify your number 1 stressor, you need to keep a log for a week, noting when you feel stressed and what you think is causing the stress. Also log any stress symptoms such as headaches, muscle tension, or inadequate time for necessary tasks.
- To add stress stimulation or challenge: Join an organized group (club). Go to a social event such as a dance or barbecue. Introduce yourself to someone new in your classes. Take on a new responsibility by becoming an officer in a club, a baby-sitter, or a part-time or volunteer worker. Take a heavier course load. Become a tutor.

Maintainer

- Make a plan for how you will handle the added stressors of special events such as traveling, holidays, registration, oral presentations, and final examinations.

· Learn another stress management strategy so that if you need it in the future you will be ready to use it. (Maybe try something in the action taker list that you are not already doing.)
· Continue to develop healthy relationships with others.

ADDITIONAL STUDENT ACTIVITIES

Activity 11.1 What's Your Personality Type? (page 261)

LABS

Lab 11.1 What Can I Do? (pages 271–272)
Lab 11.2 The Distress-Eustress Continuum (pages 273–274)
Lab 11.3 How Do I Spend My Time (page 275)

RESOURCES

Suggested Reading

American Heart Association, Greater Long Beach Chapter. Stress—bona fide A.H.A. risk factor. *Heart Lines* 41:1 February, 1984.

Cortell, R. R. *Stress management.* Guilford, CT: The Dushkin Publishing Group, 1992.

Crews, D., and D. Landers. A meta-analytic review of aerobic fitness and reactivity to psychosocial stressors. *Medicine and Science in Sports and Exercise* 19: 5114-5120, 1987.

DeLongis, A., J.C. Coyne, G. Dakof, S. Folkman, and R.S. Lazarus. Relationships of daily hassles, uplifts, and major life events to health status. *Health Psychology* 1:119-136, 1982.

Hobfoll, S.E. *Stress, social support and women.* Washington, D.C.: Hemisphere Publishing, 1986.

International Society of Sport Psychology. *Physical Activity and Psychological Benefits*: Position Statement 20: 179, 1992.

Matheny, K.B., and R.J. Riodan. *Stress and Strategies for Lifestyle Management.* Atlanta: Georgia State University, Business Press, 1992.

Morse, D.R., and M.L. Furst. *Stress for success.* New York: Van Nostrand Reinhold, 1979.

Murphy, L.R., and T.F. Schoeborn. *Stress Management in Work Settings.* New York: Praeger, 1989.

Newman, J. *How to Stay Cool, Calm, and Collected.* New York: American Management Association, 1992.

Selye, H. *The stress of life*, 2nd ed. New York: McGraw Hill, 1976.

Stanford, S.C., and P. Salmon, eds. and J.A. Gray, consultant, ed. *Stress from synapse to syndrome*. San Diego: Academic Press, 1993.

Organizations

American Association of Therapeutic Humor
222 S. Meramec
Suite 303
St. Louis, MO 63105
Tel: (314) 863-6232
Fax (314) 863-6457
Web site: http://ideanurse.com/aath

American Institute of Stress
124 Park Avenue
Yonkers, New York 10703
Tel: (914) 963-1200
Fax: (914) 965-6267
Web site: http://www.stress.org

Video

How Well Do You Manage Stress?
YMCA Program Store, Box 5077
Champaign, IL 61820

Creating and Maintaining Healthy Relationships

Chapter 12

CHAPTER SUMMARY

Healthy relationships are a vital part of wellness because they affect both quality and quantity of life. Such relationships require unconditional love, understanding, and selflessness. Healthy relationships can take on a variety of forms, all of which have love at their center. Physical intimacy is only a part of long-lasting relationships; in order to succeed, partners must also be able to communicate effectively, fight fairly, forgive, and forget. Participating in healthy relationships increases personal happiness and may reduce the risk of illness.

LEARNING OBJECTIVES

A student will be able to:
- define and describe a healthy relationship.
- explain why healthy relationships are important to total wellness.
- describe the three phases of social maturity.
- delineate the role of a good friend.
- discuss the pros and cons of marriage.
- describe the characteristics of a healthy marriage.
- describe the characteristics of a healthy family.
- identify the physical and social disadvantages of loneliness.
- determine the health of his/her own personal relationships.
- identify behaviors to maintain or change that result in healthy relationships.

PERSONAL PROFILE

Paul Newman and Joanne Woodward: A Lifelong Relationship

In the fast-paced lifestyles of Hollywood's most popular stars, it is rare for marriages to last for more than just a few years. But right in the middle of the marriage and divorce roller coaster that is so common to Hollywood, there is one relationship that has passed the test of time.

For more than 35 years Paul Newman and Joanne Woodward have demonstrated what it takes to successfully overcome the many trials and tribulations that so often destroy marriages, especially those made in Hollywood. Their marriage began in 1958 when they were both starring in the Southern melodrama, The Long Hot Summer. Both enjoyed successful acting careers, but Paul's popularity quickly catapulted him to the forefront of Hollywood's elite. Stardom was also one of Joanne's career goals, but she was not so fortunate, and her struggle to reach the top almost destroyed their relationship. The constant strain of trying to be a mother to their three daughters and have a stellar acting career was too much to handle. She calls the impossible expectation for women to "have it all," to stay thin, glamorous, and healthy, to raise a family, and to keep a career flourishing "the tough fight." Over the years, Joanne came up with elaborate ways to try to keep her identity from being overwhelmed by the huge amount of attention her husband received—mostly from women. During these difficult times, Paul and Joanne pulled together rather than apart. They have tended to their relationship, by putting it first often enough to keep it going. And, somehow, they have emerged through all the turbulence still in love.

By pulling together to overcome differences, Paul and Joanne are likely to continue their marriage for many years to come. Amid Hollywood's constant social and emotional pressure, it is refreshing to see a relationship span a lifetime.

From Paul Newman and Joanne Woodward. A lifetime of shared passions, by Maureen Dowd, *McCalls*, January, 1991, 78-82, 127, used with permission.

CONTENT OUTLINE

I. Healthy relationships support emotional, mental, and social wellness.
    A. The lack of healthy relationships can result in social isolation, depression, loneliness, and low self-esteem.
    B. All human beings have the need for intimacy; the need to give and receive.
    C. Healthy relationships include friendships as well as the union formed between couples.
    D. Close personal communication plays a key role in healthy relationships.
    E. Closeness may involve emotional, spiritual, or physical intimacy—sometimes all three.
II. An intimate relationship is one that has a high degree of closeness in the form of a friendship, relationship or association.
    A. There are intimate relationships that do not include physical intimacy.
        1. two people can have an intimate intellectual association if they share and discuss personal and deep intellectual ideas
        2. two people can share an emotional intimacy after sharing an intensely stressful situation
    B. Intimacy includes love, trust, kindness, respect, communication, etc.
    C. Human sexuality in a healthy relationship allows individuals to experience mature feelings of love, kindness, selflessness, and complete trust.
    D. Human sexuality improperly used can destroy a relationship, lead to distrust, heartache, and possibly physical disease.
III. Stages of maturity
    A. Selfishness
        1. thinking only of one's own needs and wants
        2. natural part of a young person's life (baby crying for needs, etc.)
        3. during childhood children begin to tolerate the idea that they won't always get what they want, even if they don't understand why

           4.   some people never get beyond this stage; their happiness depends on getting what they want

   B.   Learned tolerance

        1.   transition from selfishness to learned tolerance is usually long, difficult and painful

        2.   often demonstrated by adolescents

        3.   teens learn to accept and follow rules even if they don't always understand the reasons behind the rules

        4.   accept that they will not always get what they want

   C.   Selflessness

        1.   ability to put someone else first

        2.   "give and take" relationships rather than "take and take"

        3.   allows for the development of true happiness, love, empathy, joy, and compassion

        4.   these kinds of relationships enhance a person's quality of life

IV.   Healthy relationships and wellness

   A.   Social support is a key factor in protecting health.

        1.   supportive friends and family help buffer against stress-related illness and premature death

        2.   the effect that a network of close personal relationships can have on someone suffering from life's major stresses is sometimes called a "safety net"

   B.   Friendships

        1.   true friends provide value and a sense of self-worth to both parties

            a.   provide unconditional love

            b.   accept faults and weaknesses without being judgmental or critical

            c.   most long term friendships are formed in adolescence

            d.   lasting friendships require an investment of trust, acceptance, support and intimacy

        2.   men and women express friendship differently

            a.   women tend to

                (1)   talk and listen to each other using more expressive communication

                (2)   offer support and understanding

                (3)   be more tactile (hugs, etc.)

            b.   men tend to

                (1)   do things together rather than talk

                (2)   may use touch but usually only as a pat on the back

            c.   both genders will joke about problems with close friends because they feel secure; there is an unspoken code of acceptance

        3.   trust grows as confidences are shared and confidentiality kept

        4.   suggestions for nurturing friendship:

            a.   appreciate your friends and let them know

            b.   confide in your friends; it shows trust

            c.   be willing to share material things

            d.   accept your friend's mistakes and shortcomings

            e.   spend time together

   C.   Dating

        1.   any social occasion shared by two individuals (lovers, friends, or total strangers)

2.   it is a time to meet new friends. lovers. and potential mates
3.   difficult time in life because interacting with others can be everything from confusing, exhilarating, and terrifying—an emotional roller coaster
4.   physical attraction is often the main reason two people date
5.   for a relationship to develop, more than physical attraction is needed
6.   dating is a time for learning more about the other person, and the dating relationship can act as a barometer for married life

D.   Marriage
    1.   90% of Americans will marry sometime in their lives
    2.   natural extension of a trusting, sharing, loving, committed relationship
    3.   should provide unconditional support and love
    4.   offers legal and financial benefits as well as the opportunity to pool resources
    5.   limits risk of sexually transmitted diseases if the relationship remains monogamous
    6.   provides the basis for a family; support for children
    7.   happily married people experience greater health benefits; in general they experience less illness and disease and recover more quickly when they do become ill than unmarried individuals
       a.   live longer than those who are unmarried
       b.   married men are less prone to alcoholism, accidents, and illness
       c.   divorced. widowed, and single people are more likely to die of heart disease and to have weaker immune systems
    8.   people in unhappy marriages do not experience any added health benefit and actually die earlier
       a.   body reacts to conflict with changes in the immune system, including high blood pressure. hormone changes, and the stress response
       b.   marriage in and of itself may not influence health; the protective effect may be the result of the quality of a relationship
       c.   signs of trouble—think twice before marrying if:
          (1)   you and your partner constantly argue
          (2)   you and your partner feel pressured to marry because of pregnancy
          (3)   your partner wants to change you
          (4)   you want to change your partner before or after marriage
          (5)   friends or family have misgivings
          (6)   you are both young (under age twenty)
    9.   marriages tend to do well when couples:
       a.   have realistic expectations. especially about each other
       b.   argue or fight fairly (see Table 12.1)
          (1)   couples who learn to fight fairly have a 50% lower divorce rate
          (2)   fair fighting reduces likelihood of physical violence
          (3)   fair fighting teaches children how to handle disagreements
       c.   manage money well
          (1)   spending money for both spouses regardless of his/her working status
          (2)   setting financial goals together and living within one's means
       d.   set priorities

             (1)   balancing needs of the couple, children, and careers while considering each other's opinions and desires

             (2)   equal input into important decisions

E.   Family

    1.   is the fundamental unit of society; within the confines of the family, children learn the values and behaviors that they will carry into adult life

        a.   love and respect

        b.   rejection and abuse

    2.   family structure has changed over the past few decades

        a.   traditional families have a working father, homemaker mother and children

             (1)   less than 10% of the population lives in a traditional family

        b.   single-parent families are increasing

             (1)   a single-parent home that is loving and nurturing can be as successful raising children as a traditional home

             (2)   more difficult because of added financial burdens and no one to share homemaker chores and time with children

             (3)   number of one-parent homes will double by the year 2000

             (4)   since 1960, number of divorces, births to unwed parents, and teen pregnancies has more than quadrupled

             (5)   more than 50% of children can expect to spend at least one year living in a single-parent home before the age of 18

    3.   family violence occurs across all segments of society: rich and poor, rural and urban, and across all races

        a.   family violence is about demonstrating power dominance

             (1)   it includes spouse-battering, sexual abuse and marital rape, and child abuse and neglect

             (2)   can occur between parents, parent and child, siblings, and against elderly relatives

             (3)   can be physical or psychological

             (4)   violent events are often preceded by a predictable cycle of events

                  (a)   avoidance so as not to provoke the other person

                  (b)   period where grievances are internalized instead of expressed

                  (c)   accumulated grievances erupt into violence

                  (d)   period of conciliation and remorse

             (5)   counseling is usually required to break a pattern of violence

V.   Troubled relationships

    A.   Just the consideration of ending a relationship is a sign that the relationship is in trouble

    B.   Poor relationships may suffer from:

        1.   poor communication

            a.   communication breakdowns may be subtle and go unnoticed until emotional confrontation brings them to attention

            b.   either partner may stop listening or cease to be emotionally present

            c.   results in feelings of being unwanted, ignored, unappreciated

            d.   partner(s) seeks validation elsewhere

        2.   a lack of time spent together

           a.   grow apart

           b.   find more reward in spending time with others

        3.   physical, sexual or emotional abuse

           a.   should not be tolerated; if the abuser won't change, terminate the relationship

           b.   punishable by law

           c.   if not stopped, the cycle of abuse will be passed on to children

           d.   demeaning, hurtful and immoral

           e.   counseling may be effective

    C.   Relationships in trouble can seek help from marriage counselors, support groups, religious and social organizations.

VI.   Terminating a relationship can be a very painful and difficult experience.

    A.   In some cases, it is the right thing to do (especially when there is abuse).

    B.   Emotional scars for adults and children can last for years (especially in divorce cases).

    C.   Each year at least 1 million marriages end in divorce.

VII.   Living single

    A.   The number of living single adults has been increasing over the past few decades

        1.   due in part to the increased number of divorces, people staying single longer before marrying, and elderly women who outlive their husbands

        2.   surveys indicate that most singles would prefer to marry but have not yet had the right opportunity

    B.   About 37% of the U.S. population is single at any given time including:

        1.   young people who have not yet married

        2.   divorced adults

        3.   widows and widowers

        4.   homosexual partners who cannot legally marry

        5.   others who choose to be single

VIII.   Loneliness occurs when current social relationships fall short of ideal, or when the social network surrounding a person becomes deficient in quality or quantity.

    A.   Happens to single and married individuals.

    B.   Affects self-esteem and sense of self-worth.

        1.   may lead to depression, anxiety, or physical illness

        2.   may require professional help to regain social wellness

    C.   May lead to substance abuse when a person's best friend is a drug, alcohol or tobacco.

    D.   Research shows strong correlation between loneliness and premature death and illness.

        1.   increased risk of heart disease

        2.   decreased immune function

        3.   cancer

        4.   shortened life span

        5.   one study found a greater probability for suicide, mental illness, and malignant tumors

        6.   relationship of loneliness and disease remains strong even when variables like poverty, previous illness and age are accounted for

    E.   Loneliness can be cured by building social contacts and support.

        1.   for difficulties making and keeping close relationships consult a parent, professional counselor, or religious leader

2. to meet others, consider joining a church or synagogue, club, or support group

BEHAVIOR BOOSTS: STAGE-BASED STUDENT ACTIVITIES

Precontemplator
- Making good friends takes time. Think about someone with whom you would enjoy a friendship.
- Look closely at the people in your life. Do any of them enjoy a healthy relationship? If so, are they happy? Why?

Contemplator
- Imagine yourself enjoying a healthy relationship. How would your life be different?
- Give someone your undivided attention and see how he or she reacts.
- Review the box "How to Be a Good Friend" in this chapter and think about your relationships with your closest friends.

Preparer
- Stop talking and listen
- Spend time with someone.
- Say "I love you" to someone you really care about.
- Do one act of kindness for a friend or family member.

Action Taker
- Give as much of yourself as you can give to the people who mean the most to you; your relationship will get even better.
- When you fight, fight fairly and always make up afterward (see the box "Fighting Fairly" in this chapter).
- Admit it when you are wrong.

Maintainer
- Call someone you've been thinking of.
- Perform a random act of kindness. Cook supper for a neighbor, help someone in need, or do something really nice for someone you really like.

ADDITIONAL STUDENT ACTIVITIES

Activity 1: What Are Your Expectations For Marriage?

Evaluate your expectations of marriage using the questionnaire in Activity 12.1 on page 282.

Activity 2: A Letter to a Friend

Learning to communicate effectively is essential for developing healthy relationships with other people. At the beginning of this chapter, you indicated a relationship you would like to think about with regard to the material presented in this chapter. This lab gives you an opportunity to write a personal letter to the person you have been thinking about (or another person, if you prefer). As you write your letter, try to express your feelings about the relationship you have with the other person in an honest manner. The entire letter does not have to discuss how you feel about the person, but your feelings should come across in some way. You may or may not choose to send this letter.

When you have finished your letter, read through it and underline three or four main points in the letter. Which of these points have you previously conveyed to the person? Which of these points have you not previously expressed? Draw a star by the ones you haven't shared.

Why have you not expressed these feelings in the past?

How could you impart to the other person each of the points you starred?

Make a commitment to effective communication between you and the other person. Begin by selecting one of the items you starred and determining a time in the next two weeks when you will share your feelings with that person. When would an appropriate time be?

Activity 3: Understanding Your Family by Exploring Family Stories

Most people leave their family of origin with a corpus of "received stories" that have become their taken-for-granted assumptions about themselves, their ideals, and the workings of the world. Through courtship stories, birth stories, and survival stories, we are recruited into the family values that are central to our society. If and when we begin to question some of the taken-for-granted assumptions of our stories, we enter a transformative stage of life in which we can take control of our stories and stand apart from, while still being a part of, our families.

Select one of the following to begin exploring your family stories:

1. Think about or write out the story surrounding your birth and first months of life. If you do not know the story or are not sure about some of the details, ask someone in the family to tell you. If you are adopted, you might prefer to explore the story of your adoption. What does this story tell you about your identity and your place in the family?

2. Ask one of your parents to tell you the story of their courtship. What does the story tell you about your parents and their relationship? What influence do you think their courtship story has had on the family?

3. Describe a survival story of your family's—a story that separates "them" from "us" or one that tells of the family overcoming hard times, adversity, suffering, or tragedy. What does the story say about your family and their values? What have you learned from this story?

Adapted from Yerby, J., N. Buerkel-Rothfuss, and A.P. Bochner. *Understanding family communication.* 2nd ed. Scottsdale, AZ: Gorsuch Scarisbrick, 1995, 214.

Activity 4: Family Traits

Below is a list of traits common to successful families. Before looking at these traits try to think of traits that describe your family and/or a successful family you know.

Although there is a tremendous amount of variation between families, successful families share the following characteristics. As you read these, think about how you might be able to incorporate them into your family if they aren't already a part of family life.

- Many families believe it is important to spend time doing things together. The activity itself is not important as long as each family member feels important and wanted. What family activities does your family do?

- Successful families share common values. If there are differences in values, confusion and conflict may result as children try to determine for themselves what is right or wrong. Having similar spiritual beliefs may provide great emotional and social strength as families come together during hard times. What values do you share as a family or differ on?

- During hard times healthy families are not afraid to seek help from others including clergy, counselors, psychologists, social workers, or professionals. Recognizing that help is needed and taking steps to get that help is a sign that the family wants to stay together. During difficult times how did/does your family cope?

- The parents of healthy families are faithful to each other . Nothing will destroy a marriage or family faster than failure to remain true and committed to maintaining sexual fidelity. As far as you know, have your parents been faithful to each other? If not, how did the family deal with infidelity?

- Communication in healthy families always goes two ways. Parents and children effectively listen and talk through problems and difficulties. Fighting still occurs, but peaceful and fair compromises are found for disagreements and problems, and there is an increased outpouring of love after the disputes have ended.

- Do you feel like your family listens to you? Do you listen to and value your family's input? When you disagree, does it result in a rift or does the issue get resolved?

- Home for successful families is a happy place where children want to be. It is a place where everyone feels welcome and comfortable. Is your home an emotionally safe and happy place? Do you look forward to going home?

Activity 5: Maintaining Friendship at a Distance

Do you have a long-distance friendship? If so, which of the following strategies do you use to maintain it?

_____ Call at least once a week.   _____ Write letters.

_____ Call at least once a month.   _____ Visit weekly.

_____ Communicate by electronic mail at least weekly.   _____ Visit monthly.

_____ Call once or twice a year.   _____ Visit occasionally.

Now, identify three ways you might strengthen the closeness between you and a friend.

1. _____

2. _____

3. _____

Adapted from Wood, J.T. Everyday encounters: An introduction to interpersonal communication. Wadsworth, Belmont, CA, 1996.

Activity 6: Your Friendship Style

Do gender dynamics operate in your friendships with members of the same gender? Find out by completing this activity.

Think about how you relate to your closest friends of the same gender. Read the different activities listed below. Circle the number in front of each of the things you commonly do with these friends.

1. Talk about family problems.
2. Exchange favors (provide transportation, lend money)
3. Engage in sports, including shooting hoops and so forth.
4. Try to take their minds off problems with diversions.
5. Disclose your personal anxieties and fears.
6. Talk about your romantic relationships.
7. Do things together (camping, going to a game, shopping).
8. Confide secrets you wouldn't want others to know.
9. Just hang out without a lot of conversation.
10. Talk about small events in your day-to-day life.
11. Provide practical assistance to help friends.
12. Talk explicitly about your feelings for each other.
13. Discuss and work through tensions in your friendship.
14. Physically embrace or touch to show affection.
15. Ignore or work around problems in the friendship.

Items 1, 5, 6, 8, 10, 12, 13, 14 have been found to be more prominent in women's friendships.
Items 2, 3, 4, 7, 9, 11, and 15 tend to be more pronounced in men's relationships.

Adapted from Wood, J.T. Everyday encounters: An introduction to interpersonal communication. Wadsworth, Belmont, CA, 1996.

LABS

Lab 12.1 What Can I Do? (pages 287–291)
Lab 12.2 How Healthy Is Your Relationship? (pages 290–291)

RESOURCES

Suggested Readings

Christen, B.J. *Utopia against the family: The problems and politics of the American family.* New York: Ignatius Press, 1990.

Gottman, J., C. Notarius, J. Gonso, and H. Markman. *A couple's guide to communication.* Champaign, IL: Research Press, 1976.

Lederer, W.J., and D. Jackson. *The mirages of marriages.* New York: W.W. Norton, 1968.

Miller, S., D. Wackman, E. Nunnally, and C. Saline. *Straight talk.* New York: New American Library, 1982.

Scarf, M. *Intimate partners.* New York: Random House, 1987.

Tannen, D. *You Just Don't Understand.* New York: Ballantine Books, 1991.

Organizations

Emotional Health Anonymous
2420 San Gabriel Blvd.
Rosemead, CA 91770

See also Chapter 14 for drug and alcohol support groups.

Additional Local and Community Resources

Local therapists and counseling organizations

Preventing Sexually Transmitted Diseases

Chapter 13

CHAPTER SUMMARY

Sexually transmitted diseases (STDs) are uncomfortable and sometimes deadly diseases, only some of which are curable, and all of which are preventable. As long as individuals engage in unprotected sexual activity with infected partners, STD incidence will continue to increase, in some cases to epidemic levels. Although scientists are struggling to find better treatments, the best way to stop the spread of STDs is through responsible low-risk behavior. Changing risky sexual behaviors is often a difficult task. Good communication within a relationship enhances the chances of engaging in safer sex or postponing sex until both partners are comfortable and protected from disease. Prevention of disease includes abstinence or a monogamous relationship, and use of a latex condom with spermicide. Prevention also includes avoiding multiple partners, unprotected sex, mixing sex with alcohol and drugs, and avoiding contaminated needles or contact with bodily fluids of an infected person. Persons who have engaged in sexual contact that may have put them at risk for a disease need to have a medical check-up as early as possible as early detection aids in the treatment of STDs.

LEARNING OBJECTIVES

The student will be able to:
- define the terms "sexually transmitted disease" and "safer sex."
- identify the common methods of transmission of STDs.
- recognize the signs and symptoms common to most STDs.
- identify risky sexual behavior and the potential consequences.
- assess personal risk of disease using demographic and personal choice factors.
- identify steps a person can take to diminish or eliminate the risk of contracting or passing on an STD.
- discuss the role that relationship skills, especially communication skills, play in STD management and safer sex.
- discuss STDs in terms of race and gender.
- distinguish between bacterial, viral, protozoan, and parasitic diseases and their treatments.
- identify methods that do and do not transmit HIV.
- explain the relationship between HIV and other STDs.

PERSONAL PROFILE

The Faces of HIV and AIDS

AIDS is a preventable disease when precautions are taken and loved ones are informed of their risk. With more funds being made available for AIDS research there is new understanding of the virus, and effective ways to treat it are being developed. However, a cure still appears to be many lives away. Compassion, fortunately, can come more quickly. No one deserves this disease. Here are just a few of the many faces of AIDS.

Arthur Ashe

Arthur Ashe (1943–1993), one of the greatest professional tennis players of all time, became Wimbledon Champion in 1975 when he defeated Jimmy Connors. Injured late in his career, Ashe fought his way back into the top ten, only to have a heart attack at age thirty-six. He subsequently retired from competition in 1980 and put his energy into becoming a writer, broadcast journalist, and political activist. Throughout his career, Ashe, the epitome of good sportsmanship, generosity, and commitment, was an outstanding role model to all children and especially to African-American young people. He was the first Black to win a major men's tennis tournament and worked hard to bring the game of tennis to Black communities. Undergoing a second bypass operation in 1983, Ashe became infected with HIV through a blood transfusion. A very private man, Ashe was extremely upset when a reporter found out and was going to publish his story. Arthur went public on his own and let it be known that he would not be a pawn for the activist agenda. However, he decided to think about what he might do to raise AIDS awareness. He became an active fund-raiser and speaker on behalf of AIDS research and co-authored the book, Days of Grace: A Memoir. Arthur Ashe died in 1993.

Ryan White

Ryan White, born in Indiana, was only nine years old when he contracted the AIDS virus through a blood transfusion for his hemophilia. When he was diagnosed with HIV, Ryan was banned from attending public school and was ostracized by the community. Some claimed that Ryan was spitting on their children's food in an effort to infect them. Realizing they were the victims of an uneducated public, the Whites moved to another town where people were more accepting. Ryan eventually became a spokesperson for AIDS, traveling the country to speak to young people about AIDS, about his feelings, and about safer sex. He even appeared on the Phil Donohue show. In 1990, Ryan White died at age 18. His mother, along with many others, lobbied Congress to pass a bill that would provide funding that would help other AIDS patients, especially the young. The Ryan White Care Act was passed in 1990 and was renewed in 1995.

Mary Fisher

Mary Fisher is a wife, mother, author, and artist. In 1991, at the age of 40, the life she had worked so hard to build came tumbling down when she tested positive for HIV. She had been infected by her former husband (who probably contracted it through drug abuse) during their marriage. The mother of two boys (one biological and one adopted), she then waited in agony for the results of an HIV test for her biological son. To her great relief, Max tested negative. In her autobiography, My Name is Mary, Mary writes of the pain of losing contact with her biological father, of living through her mother's battle with alcohol and then her own, the pain of her own divorce, and her present AIDS journey.

Her mother remarried when Mary was four, to one of the most influential men in America, Max Fisher. Mary grew up in a privileged home, surrounded by loving relatives and visited by many famous and powerful figures. By her own admission, she struggled to find her own identity—to be something other than Max Fisher's daughter. She became a television producer and then the first woman to be an "advance man for the White House," and finally discovered her niche as an artist. Her marriage had ended, but she was finally feeling in control of her life when suddenly AIDS changed everything.

Mary has found a new mission in her role as spokesperson for AIDS. Because of her family's political connections, her previous work in fund raising, and her job as an "advance man" for President Ford, she has access to people with the power to help the AIDS movement. In 1992 when Mary spoke at the Republican National Convention, the entire hall grew quiet, and by the end of her thirteen-minute speech many were in tears, including her father. Following is an excerpt of her speech, emphasizing the point that the disease does not discriminate and that all those infected, regardless of how they became infected, deserve compassion and help.

> "The AIDS virus is not a political creature. It does not care whether you are a Democrat or Republican. It does not ask whether you are Black or White, male or female, gay or straight, young or old. Tonight I represent an AIDS community whose members have been reluctantly drafted from every segment of American society. Though I am White, and a mother, I am one with a Black infant struggling with tubes in a Philadelphia hospital. Though I am female, and contracted this disease in marriage, and enjoy the warm support of my family, I am one with the lonely gay man sheltering a flickering candle from the cold wind of his family's rejection."

In addition to her autobiography, Mary is the author of two collections of speeches, I'll Not Go Quietly and Sleep With the Angels.

Magic Johnson

Magic Johnson was considered one of the greatest point guards and play makers in the history of the National Basketball Association (NBA). He helped lead the Los Angeles Lakers to five NBA championships between 1980 and 1989 and was the first rookie ever named most valuable player (MVP) of the NBA Finals, an award he won again in 1982 and 1987. He was also named NBA's MVP three times (1987, 1989, 1990). Magic Johnson had tremendous crowd appeal and has brought a lot of fan interest to the game of basketball.

In November of 1991 Magic Johnson announced that he had tested positive for HIV and was retiring from basketball. He believed at that time that it was in the best interest of his own health and that of his peers. In 1992 Magic made cameo appearances, first at the 1992 NBA All-Star Game and then on the 1992 Barcelona Olympic Dream Team that won gold, but when he tried to make a comeback in the fall of 1992, the fears of some outspoken NBA players forced him to call it off. He became head coach of the Lakers late in the 1993 season, but retired at the end of the season. Three years later Magic decided to return to active play. This dramatic comeback was made possible by the fact that AIDS education and research have come a long way. Most of the players who once feared they would contract AIDS from him spoke out to support Magic's decision to play. Overnight, Magic was transformed from a spokesperson on how to avoid AIDS, to a model of how to live with AIDS. He is an inspiration to many in the AIDS community.

As the result of a routine physical examination for insurance purposes, Magic Johnson received the news that he had tested positive for HIV. Johnson admits to having numerous casual sexual relations prior to marrying his long-time sweetheart Cookie. The HIV news arrived two months after their marriage and just after confirming that Cookie was pregnant. Magic was personally devastated, but he was even more concerned about the health of his wife and their unborn child. Fortunately, both his wife and baby tested negative.

In his role as spokesperson for AIDS awareness and prevention, Magic established a foundation to promote AIDS research, and wrote a book titled What You Can Do to Avoid AIDS. In his book he writes:

> "But if I had known what I do now when I was younger, I would have postponed sex as long
> as I could, and I would have tried to have it the first time with somebody that I knew I wanted
> to spend the rest of my life with. I certainly want my children to postpone sex. Now the rest
> of my life may be a lot shorter than I thought it was going to be and I may not be around to see
> my son, Andre, grow up and to see what happens to the baby Cookie and I are having in the
> summer of 1992, and, of course, I may not have the long life I want with Cookie."

Magic Johnson is now retired from basketball. He and Cookie have added to their family through adoption. Magic continues to live with the AIDS virus.

References:

Ashe, A., and A. Armpersad. *Days of grace: A memoir*, New York: Knopf, 1993.

Fisher, M. *My name is Mary*. New York: Scribner, 1996, p.240.

Johnson, E. *What you can do to avoid AIDS*. New York: Time Books, 1992.

Wulf, S. As if by magic: After years of exile, Magic Johnson is back to show the world how to live with the AIDS virus. *Time Magazine* 147(7), February 12, 1996.

CONTENT OUTLINE

I. Sexually transmitted diseases (STDs) are preventable, treatable, and sometimes curable.
- A. Prevention means abstinence, or safer sex.
  1. safer sex is defined as all the actions needed to help prevent the transmission of an STD or conception of an unwanted pregnancy
  2. people's belief systems influence sexual behavior
  3. drugs, alcohol and unhealthy relationships can result in risky behavior
- B. A responsible relationship may involve:
  1. abstaining from sex
  2. postponing sex
  3. talking about sex and sexual history
  4. using a condom or other barrier protection
  5. getting a medical examination

II.   What are sexually transmitted diseases (STDs)?
    A.   They are diseases that are passed from one person to the next through sexual contact.
        1.   as of 1989 STDs had infected an estimated 12 million people in the United States
        2.   86 percent between the ages of 15 and 29
    B.   More than 50 organisms and syndromes are recognized as being involved in sexually transmitted diseases.
    C.   Most STDs are caused by bacteria or viruses.
        1.   bacteria are microscopic organisms that can live inside the body and cause infection
            a.   bacterial STDs include syphilis, gonorrhea, chlamydia
            b.   can usually be treated and cured, especially when treatment is early
        2.   viruses are submicroscopic organisms that can grow and multiply inside living cells and cause infection
            a.   viral STDs include HIV, herpes II, hepatitis B, HPV/genital warts
            b.   are treatable, but are not curable, therefore they can recur or progress
            c.   can be transmitted through sexual and nonsexual means (e.g., injection needles)
    D.   After being infected with an STD people may remain asymptomatic (free of symptoms) for periods ranging from days to several months
        1.   during this period people can transmit the infection to others
        2.   people at risk for STDs should regularly seek an STD risk assessment including a physical examination and laboratory test to detect infections
    E.   When symptoms do appear, they typically include one or more of the following:
        1.   burning or pain during urination or defecation
        2.   itching or burning around the genitals
        3.   mucus discharge or bleeding from the genitals
        4.   ulceration or blistering
        5.   rashes on the body
        6.   flu-like symptoms
    F.   STD infection can also lead to a variety of other illnesses, including pelvic inflammatory disease (PID), cancer and death.

III. Honest communication about STDs is a vital part of the prevention and management of STDs.
    A.   A sexual partner may or may not be aware that he or she has an infection.
    B.   Steps that can be taken toward establishing a trusting, caring sexual relationship include:
        1.   talking to one another about your sexual history and concerns
        2.   having a medical checkup
        3.   looking for outward signs of disease
        4.   remember you are the one making the decision about your own health
    C.   A healthy relationship can handle honest communication.

IV.   Personal choices and demographics determine a person's STD risk. (Demography is the statistical study of the human population.)
    A.   The demographics factors most often associated with STDs are sexual orientation, gender, and socioeconomic class.
        1.   unprotected sexually active heterosexual women and homosexual men are at an increased risk (demographically speaking)

   a. sexually receptive, meaning that when the male partner introduces infection, it is deposited inside his partner's body.

   b. this increases the disease's chance of survival.

   c. women are also at greater risk than men because they tend to be less symptomatic

  2. the structure of a women's reproductive organs make her more susceptible

   a. disease can travel up the uterus into the fallopian tubes and ultimately into the pelvic cavity

   b. hormonal changes due to menstruation may also provide the disease with a desirable environment for growth

   c. women can become pregnant and pass the disease along to the fetus in utero

  3. homosexual women have the least risk of contracting STDs, since neither partner is sexually receptive

 B. Individuals' sexual behavior and the characteristics of their social group interact to increase or diminish STD risk.

  1. a promiscuous person having sex exclusively with disease-free individuals will remain healthy

  2. a person in a monogamous relationship practicing unsafe sex with an infected person is likely to become infected

  3. urban areas are often statistically cited as high risk

   a. because of dense population

   b. high numbers of socioeconomically disadvantaged individuals

  4. STD infection is less race dependent and more class dependent

V. HIV and AIDS

 A. Human immunodeficiency virus (HIV) can damage the immune system, making it difficult for the immune system to recognize and defend against infection.

  1. T-cell count is an indication of the health of your immune system.

  2. AIDS virus kills T-cells, weakening the immune system and opening the door to opportunistic infections like PCP (pneumocystis carinii pneumonia), tuberculosis or a skin cancer known as Kaposi's sarcoma.

  3. Over one million cumulative cases of AIDS have been identified or are suspected in more than 165 countries. In 1993, it was estimated that over ten million people worldwide were infected with HIV.

 B. HIV can be transmitted whenever the internal fluids of one individual come in contact with the internal fluids of someone carrying the virus.

  1. HIV is found in blood, semen, vaginal fluids, and breast milk.

  2. During unprotected sex HIV can enter the body through tiny breaks in the tissue lining of the vagina, anus, penis, rectum and mouth.

  3. HIV can enter through cuts or sores in the skin.

  4. Sharing needles or equipment with an infected individual can also result in transmission.

 C. An HIV-positive woman has a one in four chance of passing the virus on to her child before or during birth if she receives no treatment.

  1. AZT treatments during pregnancy or labor may reduce the risk of infecting the baby to about one in twelve.

D. AIDS was first discovered in the United States in 1978.
1. Stringent tests for donated blood were established in 1985.
2. In the United States the risk of receiving HIV through a blood transfusion is now very small.
E. There are a number of misconceptions about how HIV can be transmitted.
1. You can't get it by shaking hands, hugging, or touching things an infected person has touched.
2. It is not airborne or food borne.
3. You cannot get it through everyday contact with infected people at school, work, home or anywhere else.
4. You won't get HIV from clothes, drinking fountains, phones or toilet seats.
5. It isn't passed on by things like forks, cups or other objects that someone infected with the virus has used.
6. You will not get HIV from eating food prepared by an infected person.
7. You won't get HIV from a mosquito bite.
8. You won't get HIV from contact with sweat, saliva, or tears.
9. You won't get HIV from casual or social kissing.
   a. Since 1986 the CDC has recommended couples not kiss deeply if one of the partners has the AIDS virus.
F. HIV may remain dormant for years.
1. An infected person may feel very healthy and still infect others.
2. When symptoms develop they start slowly and gradually worsen.
   a. The first stage, called the AIDS-related complex or ARC, may include swollen lymph glands or fever, night sweats, skin rashes, diarrhea, sores, weight loss and tiredness.
   b. In full blown AIDS the immune system is very weak, which allows opportunistic infections to spread.
G. In three to six months following infection the body will have produced enough HIV antibodies to be detected by a blood test.
H. There are no successful cures or vaccines for AIDS at this time; however, there are a number of antiretroviral therapies available to help manage HIV
1. The FDA has approved eleven drugs through an accelerated approval system.
2. Drug therapies require strict adherence and close management and may cost $10,000 per year.

VI. Hepatitis B
A. It is caused by the hepatitis B virus.
B. The portion of cases attributed to sexual contact between men has declined in recent years, while the proportion attributed to heterosexual contact and injection drug use has increased.
C. It is estimated that up to one half of all hepatitis B infections are sexually transmitted.
1. Multiple sex partners and high risk sex, especially receptive anal intercourse, place both gay men and heterosexual women at increased risk.
D. The disease affects the liver; the skin and eyes may turn yellow (jaundice).
1. Other symptoms include fever, nausea, and abdominal pain.
2. People with hepatitis B may develop cirrhosis, carcinomas, and chronic active hepatitis.

    E.   It can be diagnosed using a blood test.

    F.   Treatment for hepatitis B is prevention in the form of a vaccine

        1.   Health workers, teachers, and people who travel to less developed countries are all encouraged to get vaccinated.

        2.   Alcohol should be avoided as this aggravates the condition.

VII. Gonorrhea

    A.   Caused by a bacterium called Neisseria gonorrhea, usually found in the white blood cells.

    B.   One of the most commonly reported diseases in the United States with approximately 700,000 cases each year.

    C.   Transmission is through direct contact of mucus membranes during vaginal, anal or oral sexual contact

        1.   Babies can be infected during birth.

        2.   It is possible become infected repeatedly.

        3.   Condoms will block transmission from the vagina or penis, but the disease can still be spread from the mouth or anus.

        4.   Women are particularly susceptible.

            a.   it is estimated that 90 percent of women will become infected after a single episode of vaginal intercourse with an infected partner

            b.   men have a 33 percent chance of contracting the disease during a single act of vaginal intercourse with an infected partner

    D.   Eighty percent of infected women will not have symptoms, and between 10 and 30 percent of infected men will have either minor or no symptoms.

        1.   when symptoms do appear, they do so from two to ten days after exposure

            a.   both men and women may experience pain and/or burning during urination and a yellowish white or yellowish green discharge

            b.   women may mistake this discharge for a normal ovulation discharge

        2.   gonorrhea can affect the rectum, throat, tonsils, and eyes, the urethra in men and the reproductive organs in women

        3.   in women it most commonly affects the genital tract, specifically the cervix

    E.   It is the most common cause of pelvic inflammatory disease, approximately 30 to 60 percent.

        1.   Pelvic inflammatory disease (PID) occurs when infectious bacteria escapes into the pelvic cavity.

        2.   the risk of PID can be reduced:

            a.   use of oral contraceptives decreases the risk by 70 percent and barrier methods (like condoms) decrease risk by 60 percent

            b.   by delaying sexual intercourse (beyond adolescent years)

            c.   by protecting against and being screened for vaginal infections

            d.   by having fewer sex partners

    F.   In men gonorrhea most commonly infects the urethra.

        1.   men may notice swollen lymph glands in the groin along with penile discharge

        2.   damage to the penis can make urination difficult and erection impossible

        3.   epididymis (part of the scrotum) may become infected and scar tissue may block the flow of semen from the testicles

    G.   Babies' eyes can be infected during birth and cause blindness if untreated.

H. If gonorrhea spreads to the bloodstream of either gender, it can cause gonococcal arthritis of the joints, damage heart valves and affect the spinal cord or brain.

I. Lab techniques using fluid from the penile discharge are highly accurate; women are encouraged to have a culture of the cervical discharge done.

J. Gonorrhea is treated through oral antibiotics such as penicillin.

VIII. Syphilis

A. Caused by a bacterium called Treponema pallidum.

B. Transmission is from one person to another through direct contact with the sores of someone who is infected or through contact with mucus membranes during kissing, vaginal or anal intercourse or oral-genital contact

    1. bodily fluid contact between persons through a break or opening in the skin or mucus membranes can also result in infection

C. Syphilis passes through four stages if it is not treated:

    1. Primary stage: ten to ninety days after exposure, a small painless open sore or chancre develops at the entry site of the infection; it usually occurs on the shaft of the penis or around the vaginal opening.

    2. Secondary stage: two to twelve weeks after the appearance of the chancre, a nonitchy pinkish to brown rash may cover the whole body or appear in a few places like the face, hands or feet or around the genitals.

        a. may have a low grade fever, headache, malaise, swollen lymph nodes, white patches on the mucus membranes of the mouth and throat, patches of hair loss and open sores around the genitals and mouth

    3. Latent stage: the infecting bacteria continue to multiply but the individual appears to be healthy.

        a. this stage may last for one to forty years

    4. Tertiary stage, in this stage the syphilis infection that has continued to multiply attacks the brain, heart, and other organs and can be fatal

        a. victims may experience facial tremors, slurred speech, impaired vision or headaches, deafness, convulsions, heart disease, paralysis, memory loss, depression, insanity, and death

D. Antibiotics, usually penicillin, provide an effective treatment.

IX. Chlamydia

A. Caused by a bacterium called Chlamydia trachomatis.

B. It is the most widespread bacterial STD in the United States today.

    1. Infects three to five million people each year

        a. infects about 20 percent of all college students.

    2. Chlamydia frequently occurs along with gonorrheal infections.

    3. Chlamydia may also cause PID in as many as half a million women.

C. It is transmitted through direct contact of mucus membranes during vaginal and anal sexual activity.

    1. May be accidentally transmitted from the genitals to the eyes by the fingers.

    2. Mothers can transmit chlamydia to their babies during childbirth.

    3. Can be contracted repeatedly.

D. It is known as the silent STD because its early symptoms are so mild.

     1.   Fifty (50) percent of women and 25 percent of men do not experience any early symptoms.

     2.   If not diagnosed, severe damage to the reproductive organs can quietly occur.

     3.   Symptoms for women include vaginal discharge, spotting between periods, abdominal pain, burning urination and painful inflammation of the fallopian tubes.

     4.   Symptoms for men include burning on urination, testicular pain, a watery penile discharge.

         a.   responsible for half of the 500,000 cases of epididymitis (inflammation of the testicles).

            (1)   10 to 30 percent of men in this condition will become permanently sterile

E.   Chlamydia is very similar to gonorrhea, and one disease can be mistaken for the other.

     1.   Doctors can diagnose chlamydia using several tests, including examination of culture of tissue taken from the infected area

F.   When diagnosed, infections can be cured by taking tetracycline or other antibiotics.

     1.   Treatment of partners is essential to stopping the spread of chlamydia

X.   Herpes

A.   Is caused by two forms of the herpes simplex virus (HSV).

B.   HSV-1 trends to stay above the waist, causing minor health problems like cold sores.

C.   HSV-2 tends to occur below the waist and is usually known as genital herpes

     1.   HSV-2 may cause infections of the genitals and anus.

D.   As many as one in four people may be carriers of the virus.

     1.   About a half million new cases of genital herpes are reported in the United States each year.

     2.   Women are four times more likely to get the disease from men than men are to get it from women.

E.   Genital herpes is usually contracted through sexual contact with someone who has an outbreak of genital sores.

F.   Herpes is an ulcerative disease that causes painful blisters on the genitals, mouth, anus, and other mucus membranes and sometimes on the skin of other areas of the body.

     1.   Men and women infected with the herpes virus are often asymptomatic for long periods

     2.   Infected babies may develop blindness or brain damage, or even die

G.   Symptoms may appear as soon as two days or as late as thirty days after initial exposure.

     1.   The virus travels up the sensory nerve and settles in the ganglia near the spinal cord.

     2.   The virus will periodically travel back down the nerve and start multiplying near the skin again.

H.   Diagnosis is usually made through visual examination of the sores.

I.   The drug Acyclover helps heal the sores and alleviate pain, but it is not a cure.

XI.   Human Papillomavirus (HPV)

A.   Over sixty different forms of the human papillomavirus, 15 percent of which are genital warts.

B.   About 40 million people in the United States are infected with the virus, and one million new cases of genital warts are reported each year.

     1.   Some types of HPV cause genital warts which are nonulcerated and frequently recur.

        2.   Only a small percentage of HPV cases have visible warts.

        3.   Certain types of HPV are linked to precancerous lesions or cancer of the cervix, vulva, penis, anus, and throat.

    C.   The highly contagious HPV enters the skin through microscopic tears and abrasions that occur during sexual activity.

        1.   For women the cervix is the most common site of infection.

        2.   About two thirds of people who have sexual contact with an infected person will go on to develop this common STD.

    D.   Without treatment warts may spontaneously clear up, stay the same, or multiply and spread, increasing the chances of infecting others or becoming cancerous.

    E.   Diagnosis includes a Pap smear test to detect HPV infection and precancerous tissue.

    F.   There is no cure for HPV. Treatment can help manage genital warts.

        1.   After successful treatment the virus usually becomes latent or dormant.

        2.   Recurrences are possible; a person with a history of HPV should see a physician regularly.

XII.   Trichomoniasis

    A.   Caused by a parasite called trichomonas vaginalis, which is a protozoan that thrives in warm, moist places.

    B.   Trichomoniasis is one of the most common protozoan infections in the United States.

        1.   Over three million annual cases.

    C.   The primary mode of infection is sexual, though it can be transmitted nonsexually (through wet towels, bathing suits, etc.)

        1.   It is highly contagious and can be contracted repeatedly.

        2.   Men and women are equally vulnerable to this parasite and asymptomatic men represent a common pathway for reinfection of women.

    D.   Men and women with the disease may be asymptomatic for extended periods.

        1.   Symptoms for women include among others, mild to severe vaginitis, intense itching, burning, vaginal or vulvular redness, vaginal discharge.

        2.   Men are usually asymptomatic, but when symptoms do occur they consist of pus-like or watery penile drip, and pain upon urination.

            a.   Men may also experience painful swelling of the penis and/or epdidymitis.

        3.   Diagnosis is determined through microscopic examination or vaginal or penile secretions.

        4.   Oral antibiotic metronidazole (Flagyl) is 90 percent effective in curing the disease.

XIII. Candidiasis

    A.   Caused by an overgrowth of fungus that is normally present in the vagina as well as on the skin and in the mouth and digestive tract.

    B.   It is one of the most common infections of the female genital tract.

        1.   About 75 percent of women at some time in their lives experience the discomfort of a vaginal yeast infection.

    C.   Yeast infections can occur without any sexual contact or may be passed to partner through oral or genital intercourse.

        1.   An infection occurs when there is an overgrowth of the naturally occurring fungus.

            a.   can be a result of additional fungus being introduced through sexual contact

                b.   through sexual contact, use of oral contraceptives, diabetes mellitus, HIV infection, but usually the infection occurs without any of these underlying medical problems

    D.   Symptoms may include:

          1.   women: intense itching, and/or a thick cottage-cheesy discharge smelling of yeast

          2.   men: burning or itching during urination

          3.   women and men: oral contact can result in throat infection called thrush

    E.   Diagnosed through a microscopic examination of vaginal and penile discharges as well as visual examination of the vagina looking for white patches on the walls or on the vulva.

          1.   A variety of treatments may be used to treat candidiasis, the most common of which are vaginal creams and suppositories.

                a.   over-the-counter products or prescribed medicines

                b.   symptoms usually abate in a few days

    F.   To prevent infecting someone else use condoms and latex squares or remain abstinent when the infection is present.

XIV. Pubic Lice

    A.   Parasite that breeds primarily in the pubic hair.

          1.   This is a different parasite than those that cause body or head lice.

    B.   Pubic lice are transmitted through sexual contact with infected clothing, sheets, towels, or toilet seats.

          1.   Attaches itself to the skin around the genitals and lays eggs on a pubic hair shaft.

          2.   Can also migrate and be transmitted to the chest, scalp, underarm, and facial hair.

    C.   Symptoms include:

          1.   intense itching in pubic hairs, around the anus, in the armpits, and occasionally in the beard and mustache.

          2.   bites can cause a rash or small blue spots

          3.   brown specks seen in underwear

    D.   Diagnosis through examination by a clinician to identify lice and eggs attached to hairs.

    E.   Treatment: topical creams, lotions, and medical shampoos to kill the lice.

          1.   Must be eradicated from clothing, and bed linens also.

    F.   Bathing and changing underclothing every day helps prevent an infection.

XV. Relationship between HIV and other STDs.

    A.   It appears that suppressive effects of HIV on the immune system worsen the symptoms of other STDs and decreases the healing effects of STD therapies.

XVI. Avoiding STDs: Facts about prevention

    A.   The ways to protect yourself are relatively simple and few.

          1.   Abstinence or exclusive sex with a disease-free individual are the safest methods.

          2.   The next safest is use of a latex condom in combination with a spermicide.

                a.   spermicide alone is not sufficient, but it adds some effectiveness

                b.   lamb and natural skin condoms are effective for birth control but are too porous to stop many STDs, including the AIDS virus

                      (1)   the wrong lubricants can damage a condom

                      (2)   avoid oil based products like petroleum jelly, and Vaseline

          3.   It is better to take any precaution rather than none because it will reduce risk.

BEHAVIOR BOOSTS: STAGE-BASED STUDENT ACTIVITIES

Precontemplator
- Borrow the free movie on AIDS available at video rental stores
- Look at the statistics that show the high prevalence of STDs in the United States. Do you know someone who has an STD?
- Read pamphlets concerning STDs, including HIV/AIDS. These are available and free at doctors' offices, women's centers, health clinics, and many public libraries. Hotlines can also provide you with an anonymous way of locating information.
- Talk to your significant other concerning his or her feelings on abstinence, safer sex, and the prevention of disease.
- Review the pictures of the common STDs in this chapter.
- Visit or help a friend diagnosed with HIV/AIDS or another STD.
- If you travel, read about the prevalence of AIDS in other countries.
- Read through the list of symptoms for the various STDs, make a note of any symptoms you may be experiencing, and share these with your health-care provider.

Contemplator
- List your pros and cons concerning practicing abstinence or safer sex.
- List possible behaviors you would consider adopting, and consider the pros and cons to making these changes. Examples include abstinence, entering into a disease free monogamous relationship, and using protection.
- Consider getting a medical checkup to ascertain your present health status and any risk to a sexual partner.
- If you are considering using a latex condom, buy two and practice using one. This will prevent fumbling around during a romantic or passionate moment.
- Examine your spiritual beliefs concerning sexual practices and seek appropriate guidance.
- Think about the kinds of things that trigger you to have unsafe sex, such as a partner's pleas, romantic locations, or being under the influence of alcohol or drugs.

Preparer
- Get a medical checkup to ascertain your present health status and any risk to a sexual partner.
- Practice saying no to unwanted sexual contact through role playing.
- Rehearse what you want to say to your sexual partner and then make a decision when to talk to him or her.
- Sometimes people who want to abstain become tempted in certain circumstances. Think of what might tempt you and a way to avoid or handle the situation. For example, you might set a designated time to be home and have a friend call to make sure you have gotten home safely. Go to more public settings such as movies or a play. Double date with a supportive friend. Rehearse saying no. Plan how to get home by yourself if the pressure becomes too great on a date.

Action Taker
- Practice abstinence.
- Enter into a safe, monogamous relationship.

- Practice safer sex through the regular use of a latex condom.
- Check for disease on your sexual partner. Look with the lights on, watching for warts or sores and being aware of unusual odors.
- Look for needle marks or any other indication that your partner uses IV drugs.
- Discuss STD risk with any person with whom you are considering sharing sexual contact. Exchange known medical information.
- Get a medical examination to determine your present health status and any risk you present to a partner.
- If you are sexually active and already have an STD, inform your partner and practice safer sex.
- Urinate before and after sex.
- Give a pamphlet about STDs to someone you care about.
- If you are sexually active, have latex condoms readily available. Be sure that your condom is new enough to be effective and that you know how to use it. (A condom that has been in a wallet or purse too long can dry out and be easily broken.)
- Support others in their effort to practice safer sex and surround yourself with people who respect your stance.
- Make a plan for how to get out of a pressure situation and be prepared to carry it out. Examples: Rehearse saying no. Carry enough money for a phone call and a cab. Take a self-defense course. Double date with a friend and have a signal for help.

Maintainer
- Avoid situations that lead to unwanted temptation or poor judgment, such as sleeping with someone you don't know or with whom you don't intend to have sex, flirtation that leads someone to believe you are interested in sexual relations, or mixing alcohol and drugs with sex.
- If you are sexually active, purchase protection supplies ahead of time and have them readily available regardless of where and when you decide to become intimate.
- Question starting or continuing a relationship with someone who does not believe in safer sex.
- Surround yourself with people who support safer sex or abstinence.
- Renew spiritual commitments concerning sexual relations.
- If you are sexually active, you and your partner(s) should continually support and renew each other's commitment to safer sex.

ADDITIONAL STUDENT ACTIVITIES

Activity 1: STDs: Test Your Knowledge About Causes and Curability

Use Activity 13.1 on page 295 in the textbook

Activity 2: Am I at Risk for HIV?

Use Activity 13.2 on page 298 in the textbook.

Activity 3: Rank the Risk

Assuming that each of the following persons is sexually active and is not using any barrier protection, and is not involved with IV drugs, can you put them in order from highest to lowest risk for STDs? Explain why you have placed them in the order you have.

homosexual man
homosexual woman
heterosexual man
heterosexual woman

Answer Key: Lowest to Highest STD Risk

homosexual female: not exposed to ejaculate
heterosexual male: sexually insertive rather than receptive; tend to have fewer STD complications
homosexual male: sexually receptive; endemic level of disease
heterosexual female: sexually receptive; when asymptomatic there are increased risks of complications
(e.g., PID and infertility); additional risks to fetus/newborn

Activity 2: Is Your Trust Well Placed?

Note: This is a discussion activity. After reading the following, have a discussion about trust, healthy relationships, and sexual behavior.

Before trusting your physical and emotional health to someone, make sure your trust is well placed. Here is some food for thought:

Do you agree with all of these? Are they all in the same league?

- To save a friend or family member's life, I would risk my life.
- To uphold my religious values, I would lay down my life.
- To defend my country and what it stands for, I would risk my life.
- To have unprotected sex, right this minute, I would risk my life.

Before you trust someone with your wellness, ask yourself if you would trust that person to

- Hold onto $100,000 for you (or a winning lottery ticket)?
- Take car of your home? or your car?
- Back you when everyone else is against you?
- Be understanding and ready to help at 3 AM?
- Take good care of your child?
- Care for you if you became pregnant or very sick?

Consider the source. If you are being pressured into sex or to have unprotected sex, ask yourself

- How concerned is my partner about me?
- Is this the basis of a good relationship?
- Is this relationship going to last?
- Will it be good sex for me? for my partner?

Activity 3: Putting on a Condom

On separate large (8.5 x 11) placards, write each of the steps to putting on a condom. Hand out one piece of paper (step) to each student. Ask the students to line up so that the steps are in the proper order. Discuss any errors made. The following steps are in the correct order:

- Discuss Using Condoms
- Quiet Evening At Home
- Open Package
- Sexual Arousal
- Erection
- Squeeze Air Out Of Tip
- Leave Room At Tip
- Roll Condom On
- Add Lubricant (Non-O 9)
- Loss Of Erection
- Erection
- Intercourse
- Orgasm/Ejaculation
- Hold On To Rim
- Withdraw Penis
- Loss Of Erection
- Relaxation
- Dispose Of Condom

Activity 4: Spreading the Disease

Put some glitter on your hands. Shake hands with two students when they enter the room. Tell two (or more) students to refuse to shake hands with anyone in the upcoming activity. Be sure that no one overhears you telling this to the two students. Then ask the class to stand up and mingle by shaking hands with five other people and telling each of the five something interesting about themselves. Once everyone is reseated, tell the students that you "infected" two students with a disease (glitter) at the start of class. Have these two students stand. Then ask anyone else with glitter on their hands to stand. These people have also been infected. Discuss how quickly a disease can spread. Ask the two students who did not shake hands what refusal skills they used and how refusing felt. Ask others how it felt to be refused a handshake. Relate this to abstaining from sexual relations and/or practicing safer sex. At the close of this exercise make sure students understand that STDs are not spread through casual contact like a handshake. Also emphasize that it is not who we are but what we do that places us at risk for STDs.

Note: This activity can also be done using index cards upon which students collect other students signatures. The index cards can be marked using symbols that are explained later to indicate that the person holding the card used a condom, shared injection needles, abstained from sex, or had unprotected sex. A simpler method is to mark a few cards with red dots where students won't notice them and later explain that the red dot individuals are infected. Anyone who has collected the red dot person's signature is now also infected.

LABS

Lab 13.1 What Can I Do? (pages 309–311)
Lab 13.2 Safer Sex Scenarios (page 312)

RESOURCES

Suggested Reading

Biskup, M., and K. Swisher, eds. *AIDS: Opposing Viewpoints*. San Diego: Greenhaven Press, 1992.

Centers for Disease Control. *Division of STD/HIV Prevention Annual Report*, 1989. Atlanta, GA: U.S. Department of Health and Human Services, 1990.

Centers for Disease Control. 1985 STD treatment guidelines. *Mortality and Morbidity Weekly Report Supplement*, September, 1985.

Chlamydia: Cloak and dagger, *Harvard Medical School Health Letter* 13(12):7, 1988.

Donatelle, R., and L. Davis. *Brief Second Edition to Access to Health*. Prentice Hall, Englewood Cliffs, NJ, 1993.

Holmes, K.K., P.-A. Mardh, P.F. Sparling, P.J. Wiesner, W. Cates Jr., S. M.Lemon, and W.E. Stamm, eds. *Sexually transmitted diseases*, 2nd ed. New York: McGraw-Hill, 1990.

Larson, D.E., ed. *The Mayo Clinic family health book*. New York: William Morrow, 1990.

Nevid, J. *201 Things You Should Know About AIDS*. Allyn and Bacon, Boston, 1993.

Shilts, R. *And the band played on: Politics, people and the AIDS epidemic*. New York: St. Martin's Press, 1987.

U.S. Department of Health and Human Services. *Healthy people 2000: National health promotion and disease prevention objectives*. DHHS Publication No (PHS) 91-50213. Washington, D.C.: U.S. Government Printing Office, 1990.

U.S. Department of Health and Human Services. *Medicine for the public. Sexually transmitted diseases.* Public Health Service, National Institute of Health Publication No 93-3057, April, 1993.

Organizations

Center for Disease Control
Division of STD Prevention
Web site: http://cdc.gov/nchstp/dstd/dstpd

Center for Disease Control National STD Hotline
(800) 227-8922

Health Education Resource Organization
101 W. Reed Street, Suite 825
Baltimore, MD 21201

Herpes Resource Center
c/o American Social Health Associates
P.O. Box 100
Palo Alto, CA 94302
National Hotline
Tel: (919) 361-8488
    (800) 230-6039
Web site: http://sunsite.unc.edu/asha

The Kaposi's Sarcoma Foundation
520 Castro Street
San Francisco, CA 94114
(415) 864-4376

March of Dimes
National Office
1275 Mamaroneck Avenue
White Plains, NY 10605
Tel: (914) 428 - 7100
Web site: http://www.modimes.org
Planned Parenthood
Web site: http://www.plannedparenthood.org

Ryan White National Fund
c/o Athletes and Entertainers for Kids
8961 Sunset Blvd.
Los Angeles, CA 90065

San Francisco AIDS Foundation
333 Valencia
San Francisco, CA 94103
(415) 864-4376

Video

AIDS: The New Facts of Life. Newsmagazine format. Self quiz on prior knowledge and post quiz at the end. HIV, immune system, communication about sex, proper condom use. ETA Associates

Additional Local and Community Resources

State and County Health Departments (communal disease control)

Understanding and Avoiding Substance Abuse

Chapter 14

CHAPTER SUMMARY

With the growing prevalence of drugs, both legal and illegal, we have to wonder if we have become a nation that solves its problems by popping a pill, having a drink, or smoking a joint. There is plenty of evidence that we are, but there is also evidence of a growing intolerance for substance dependency. More than one Olympic athlete has been stripped of a medal because of drug use, and neighbors are joining forces to drive drug dealers out of their neighborhoods and parks. More and more people are choosing to live smoke-free, and programs like AA continue to grow as alcoholics take a stand against their addiction.

Substance abuse takes a toll in many ways. It hurts the abuser, the abuser's friends and family and is costly to society in terms of crime, rehabilitation, and lost work productivity. We can live a life that encourages health problems and then hope a wonder drug or operation will bail us out, or we can live a lifestyle that will help keep us out of the doctor's office. Baseball great Mickey Mantle became a wellness advocate following an unsuccessful liver transplant—a desperate medical attempt to solve a problem caused by excessive drinking. His message, before he died, was to live a wellness life up-front and avoid the tragedy of substance abuse.

Prevention starts with good personal decisions to avoid substance abuse. Then a proactive approach is to reach out to those near you in an effort to prevent or stop abuse. When it comes to prevention, one person can make a difference, especially when friends talk to friends, siblings talk to siblings, and parents talk to children.

LEARNING OBJECTIVES

The student will be able to:

- recognize the problems created by substance abuse and be able to discuss the impact at both a personal and societal level.
- state some of the reasons why people abuse substances.
- be able to define and give examples of abuse and addiction.
- identify the effects and risks of alcohol, tobacco, and drug abuse.
- know how and where to obtain help.
- critically review the message being presented by advertisers and pressuring peers concerning the use of certain substances.
- identify any abusive behaviors in which she or he is engaged.
- select a behavior to change or select a behavior that will help prevent substance abuse in the community.

PERSONAL PROFILE

Lobbyist Victor L. Crawford

When Victor L. Crawford was asked why he worked as a tobacco lobbyist for 6 years he said, "I did it for the money." It takes time to work your way up the ladder as a lobbyist, but when a person starts representing the big players out there, it's worth good money. Life as a lobbyist had been good for Mr. Crawford until he was diagnosed with cancer of the base of the tongue which had spread to his lungs and bones. He was told by his doctor that he had a "textbook" case of cancer caused by smoking.

Crawford started smoking cigarettes at the age of 13 and switched to a pipe and cigars in his late 30's. Until he became a cancer victim, he never really thought tobacco smoke could destroy life in such a horrible way. The tobacco industry is an extremely powerful organization which aggressively watches local, state, and national legislation with the intent of stopping any legislation which might hurt tobacco sales. Their lobbying tactics and strategies are nothing short of ruthless, which partially explains why the industry has flourished for the past 50 years.

Feeling the guilt of his efforts and the knowledge that his days were numbered, Mr. Crawford quit his job as a lobbyist and began a vigorous effort to undo the damage he and the tobacco industry had caused. He has appeared on anti-smoking TV and radio announcements. He has testified to local and state law makers in an effort to create the toughest anti-smoking bills in the nation. In short, he has done everything within his power to prevent the further loss of life. Crawford sums up his position when he states, "They (the tobacco industry) don't realize the suffering that they're causing until it happens to them, and the suffering that they're causing is beyond words."

CONTENT OUTLINE

I.   What is substance abuse?
    A.   Use of a substance even though the substance is harmful to the user or the people around the user.
    B.   A substance can be abused without a person being addicted to it.

II. What is addiction?
    A.   Addiction is an advanced form of abuse, either physical or psychological dependence.
        1.   physical dependence is characterized by tolerance to the drug and withdrawal symptoms if the level of the drug in the body drops.
        2.   psychological dependence includes an intense craving or compulsive desire for the mood-altering effects that the psychoactive ingredient in certain substances provided.
            a.   person can be psychologically dependent without being physically dependent
        3.   affects all aspects of wellness: can cloud mental judgment, interfere with or contradict spiritual beliefs, cause negative emotions and result in poor physical health

III. Why do people abuse substances?
    A.   Biological explanations
        1.   genetic predisposition and prenatal drug exposure
    B.   Psychological explanations

1.   peer pressure, family, religious influences, personal traits, social factors, such as socioeconomic background and present living conditions.
2.   people with low self esteem, who suffer from depression, or who have a tendency to take high risks are prone to addiction
3.   children of abusers are more likely to abuse substances than other children
4.   curiosity about experimentation often initiate a trip towards abuse and addiction.
5.   casual users can become abusers as the desired pleasurable effects require more and more of the abused substance

IV.   What are the costs to society?
    A.   100,000 lives are lost to alcohol; 419,000 lives to tobacco. Forty percent of all traffic fatalities and an estimated 47 to 65 percent of all drowning are alcohol related.
    B.   the expense to society is
        1.   expense of trying to prevent abuse from starting, stop on-going abuse and provide treatment for abusers.
        2.   dollars lost through a lack of productivity: employee's work is erratic, drug-related accidents , absenteeism from work, premature deaths.
        3.   expenditures for prevention education, treatment programs, health care, traffic accidents, and law enforcement.
        4.   other serious problems occur; violence, injuries, disease, rape, child and spousal abuse, AIDS, teen pregnancy, school dropouts, car crashes, escalating health care costs, low work productivity and homelessness.
        5.   1993 drug-related costs were estimated at $200 billion. $90.4 billion in health care costs alone
        6.   on campus, half of college students who were victims of campus crime said they had been drinking or using other drugs when they were victimized
        7.   alcohol is implicated in one to two-thirds of sexual assaults and acquaintance or date rape cases

V.   Substance Abuse and Behavior Change
    A.   behavior change for substance abuse can include the decisions to:
        1.   start abusing a substance
        2.   stop abusing a substance
        3.   help an abuser or potential abuser

VI.   The use and abuse of alcohol
    A.   Alcohol is tied to celebrations, religious rituals, and traditions.
    B.   Alcohol is tied to tragedy, addiction, crime, traffic accidents, spousal and family abuse.
    C.   Alcohol has innocent victims, babies born mentally retarded and disfigured, people killed by drunk drivers etc.

VII.   Alcohol is a mood altering drug that can be physically and psychologically addicting.
    A.   The psychoactive ingredient in all fermented and distilled liquors is ethyl alcohol (ethanol), that is colorless with a sharp burning taste that functions as a depressant on the central nervous system.
        1.   ethyl alcohol modifies the brain's control functions of motor coordination, reaction time, information processing, and inhibition.
        2.   the measure of how much ethyl alcohol is in a drink is known as the proof
            a.   the proof is twice the percentage of alcohol contained in the beverage
            b.   pure alcohol is 200 proof

B.   The amount of alcohol in your blood is referred to as your blood alcohol content (BAC).
    1.   most of the alcohol consumed is absorbed through the stomach (20%) and small intestine (75%) into the bloodstream
        a.   food in the stomach slows absorption
        b.   carbon dioxide (bubbles) in carbonated beverages speeds absorption
        c.   the liver extracts alcohol from the blood at a rate of about three hours for every one ounce of alcohol consumed
            (1)   drinking coffee does not speed up the process and will not sober up the person
    2.   between 3 and 10 percent of the alcohol consumed is not metabolized; instead it is excreted through the urine, breath, and sweat; basis for breath and urine BAC tests
    3.   BAC of .08 or higher is considered legally intoxicated in most states
    4.   BAC is influenced by the quantity and quality of metabolizing enzymes
        a.   women will have a higher BAC than men with the same quantity of alcohol because women metabolize alcohol more poorly due to lower amounts of alcohol dehydrogenase, a stomach enzyme that breaks down alcohol before it reaches the bloodstream
        b.   genetic differences is alcohol metabolizing enzymes have been found in certain minority groups
    5.   BAC with the same quantity of alcohol will be higher in those with a small body size and less body fat
    6.   BAC can be controlled by
        a.   what you drink
        b.   how fast you drink it
            (1)   the average male can metabolize about one drink an hour.
            (2)   binge drinking is very dangerous, putting the drinker at risk for alcohol poisoning
        c.   whether or not you eat since food slows the alcohol absorption rate

VIII. In 1956 the American Medical Association declared alcoholism a disease.
  A.   Addictive drinking follows a variety of patterns.
        a.   heavy drinking only on the weekends
        b.   large amounts daily
  B.   There is evidence of a gene that may predispose people to alcoholism.
    1.   not everybody with this gene will become an alcoholic; it means they are more susceptible to alcoholism.
  C.   Two thirds of the population drinks; only about 10 percent drink 50 percent of all the alcohol consumed in the United States.
    1.   white men and women are most likely to drink, followed by Hispanics and African-Americans.
    2.   men drink larger quantities, more frequently and report more drinking-related problems than women.
    3.   single women (unmarried, separated, or divorced) have the highest drinking rate among women
        a.   women with a history of sexual abuse are twice as likely to be problem drinkers than those without.

         4.   children of alcoholic parents are more likely to become alcoholics themselves, and these children are more likely to marry alcoholics, have an eating disorder or become involved with drugs

IX.   Effects of alcohol

    A.   Short term

        1.   alcohol depresses the brain center that controls a person's inhibition

            a.   more apt to engage in risky behavior

        2.   brain functions slow, reaction time decreases, alertness is dulled and motor coordination is impaired

            a.   dangerous to participate in activities like sports, in which quick, coordinated movements are important

        3.   judgment and the ability to reason are also affected

            a.   emotions may intensify and swing widely from one time to the next.

    B.   Long term effects

        1.   Psychological effects: paranoia, delusions, and memory gaps.

        2.   Physical effects: cirrhosis of the liver, heart disease, pancreatic inflammation, vomiting, stomach pain, nausea, digestive problems, ulcers, gastritis, brain cell damage, immune system depression; cancers, delirium tremens (muscular shakes/convulsions); malnutrition; nerve damage; menstrual irregularities; deep sleep interference; impotence; decreased vaginal lubrication; interference with body temperature regulation; increased risk of osteoporosis; increased risk of kidney disease; fetal alcohol syndrome; mental retardation; developmental delays; miscarriage

            a.   cirrhosis of the liver is the most common disease

                (1)   alcohol slows down the liver's metabolism of fats, allowing fat to accumulate in the liver cells until they burst and are replaced with fibrous scar tissue which impedes blood flow and ultimately causes liver failure and death

                (2)   women are more susceptible to liver disease because less alcohol is metabolized in the stomach, allowing more to get to the liver

    C.   Alcohol and Pregnancy

        1.   Alcohol crosses the placenta and can interrupt normal fetal development

            a.   can cause severe physical deformity, behavioral problems, clumsiness, stunted growth or mental retardation.

            b.   each year 4,000 to 12,000 babies are born with physical signs and intellectual disabilities associated with fetal alcohol syndrome..

        2.   Breast milk can pass alcohol on to the baby.

    D.   Treatment for alcohol problems

        1.   treatment starts with the individual, who must recognize the problem of alcoholism and want to do something about it

            a.   twenty-five percent of alcoholics successfully stop or reduce their drinking on their own

            b.   formal programs are available to alcoholics and members of their families

                (1)   Alcoholics Anonymous (AA): twelve step program: over 2 million members worldwide

        (2)   Rational Recovery and Secular Organizations for Sobriety (SOS); similar to AA without the same spiritual tone

        (3)   Al-teen: for young drinkers, youthful friends of drinkers, and children of alcoholics

        (4)   Al-Anon: an organization for friends and families of alcoholics.

   c.   almost 1.9 million Americans age 12 and older entered a treatment program in 1992.

   d.   18- to 34-year-olds more likely to seek treatment than those older or younger.

   e.   treatment usually includes three stages:

        (1)   detoxification

        (2)   medical treatment

        (3)   discussion and planning for long-term behavior change

   f.   withdrawal can be painful, with symptoms being

        (1)   sweating

        (2)   weakness

        (3)   delirium treatments (trembling or convulsion)

X.   The Use and Abuse of Tobacco

   A.   Tobacco products represent a major economic, political, and social force in the Untied States.

      1.   since colonial days tobacco has been one of America's largest export

      2.   today it is the seventh largest cash crop

   B.   Public opinion of tobacco has changed over the years.

      1.   1940's and 1950's movie stars glamorized smoking

      2.   1960's about half of all Americans were smokers

      3.   1964, the Surgeon General Office published its first report on the dangers of tobacco

        a.   research found increasing evidence relating tobacco use to heart disease and numerous cancers.

      4.   Anti-tobacco legislation has been successful in increasing public awareness of the dangers of tobacco use.

        a.   health risk warning on all cigarette packages and advertisements

        b.   government buildings are smoke free

        c.   about 80 percent of states have laws banning smoking in public sector workplaces.

        d.   about 30 percent of states have laws banning smoking in private sector workplaces.

        e.   Congress banned smoking on all domestic flights under six hours.

        f.   some shopping malls, restaurants and bars have become smoke free.

      5.   1995 the Surgeon General's Office labeled nicotine an addictive drug.

      6.   1997, the FDA labeled nicotine an addictive drug.

      7.   1996 President Clinton supported the FDA regulations on cigarettes which tightened access and advertising aimed at minors

      8.   today tobacco companies service over 48 million American smokers

   C.   Who smokes?

      1.   today about one-third of adults smoke and one-third of adolescents smoke.

        a.   overall adult smokers declined 40 percent between 1965 to 1990, and smoking among young people leveled off

      2.   average age for starting to smoke is thirteen, for smokeless tobacco is age ten.

3.   people who grow up around smoke are more likely to become smokers themselves.
4.   adults with less than a twelfth grade education are twice as likely to be smokers than college graduates, and high school dropouts are three times more likely to smoke.
5.   20 percent of male high school students use smokeless tobacco, nationwide 6 percent of men and 1 percent of women eighteen or older use snuff or chewing tobacco.
        (1)   sales have increased 40 percent since 1970

D.   What's in a tobacco product?
1.   the psychoactive (mood altering) drug in tobacco is an alkaloid poison called nicotine
2.   in low doses nicotine acts as a stimulant, increasing heart rate, blood pressure, alertness, the ability to concentrate and the speed at which information is processed
3.   at high dosage, nicotine acts as a sedative, reduces aggression and alleviates stress

E.   What is in a tobacco product?
1.   Nicotine enters the bloodstream either through the lungs, the membranes of the mouth or membranes of the nose; it takes only a few seconds for nicotine to reach the brain
    a.   Users will smoke or use snuff at regular intervals to maintain a level of nicotine in their blood that produces that good feeling.
    b.   If the nicotine level drops, withdrawals symptoms occur, including a strong nicotine craving
2.   Tar is made up of over 4,000 chemicals, including forty-three known to cause cancer
    a.   Tar settles in the air passages. Tar interferes with the cilia, hair like structures that normally sweep foreign particles out of the lung tissue and bronchial tubes.
3.   Carbon monoxide is a by-product of burning tobacco. When carbon monoxide is inhaled into the lungs, it preempts oxygen and readily combines with hemoglobin. As a result poorly oxygenated blood is circulated out of the body. Low levels of carbon monoxide cause shortness of breath; high levels can result in death by asphyxiation.

F.   Short term effects
1.   cigarette: smoke odor permeates surroundings, dulled sense of taste and smell
2.   snuff or chewing tobacco: bad breath, stained teeth, tooth decay, gum disease, increased blood cholesterol and dulled senses of taste and smell.
3.   tobacco products: cut down endurance, cause loss of appetite, may result in unwanted weight loss, fatigue, hoarseness, stomach pains, insomnia, diarrhea, and impaired visual acuity.
4.   nicotine may cause nausea, dizziness, clammy skin, light-headedness, rapid pulse, confusion and vomiting.

G.   Long term effects
1.   Cardiovascular disease
    a.   a majority of tobacco-related deaths are the result of cardiovascular diseases, particularly coronary heart disease (CHD).
        (1)   nearly one-fifth of deaths from cardiovascular diseases are attributable to smoking.
        (2)   smokers double their risk of heart disease and significantly increase their risk for strokes.
            (a)   tobacco substances affect the cardiovascular system by:
                i)   causing a shortage of oxygen

          ii)   promoting atherosclerosis

          iii)   forcing the heart to work harder than normal

      (b)   pulmonary heart disease occurs when the arteries feeding the lungs are affected.

      (c)   aortic aneurysm is linked to smoking.

    (3)   leg cramping, numbness and even gangrene can occur.

2.   Cancers

    a.   common cancer sites include the lips, mouth, gums, esophagus, trachea, larynx, lungs, pancreas, kidneys, colon, bladder, uterus, cervix.

      (1)   Lung cancer is the most common cancer among cigarette smokers. Mouth and throat cancer are the most common among smokeless tobacco and pipe users.

         (a)   lung cancer is twenty-three times higher for male smokers and eleven times higher for female smokers compared to people who have never smoked.

         (b)   smoking accounts for 87 percent of lung cancer and 29 percent of all cancers.

         (c)   each year 3,000 nonsmokers who work or live with smokers die of lung cancer.

3.   Chronic obstructive pulmonary disease (COPD)

    a.   emphysema and chronic bronchitis are two of the most common.

    b.   cigarette smokers are eighteen times more likely to die from COPD than non smokers.

H.   Tobacco, pregnancy, and smoking effect on children

    1.   smoking while pregnant can lead to serious complications for the newborn

    2.   nicotine, carbon monoxide, and other dangerous chemicals cross the placenta and enter the baby's body

    3.   statistics show a direct relation between smoking during pregnancy and spontaneous abortions, stillbirths, death among newborns, and sudden infant death syndrome

    4.   nicotine can be found in breast milk

    5.   smoking is suspected to impair fertility in both men and women.

    6.   children growing up around secondhand smoke experience an increased number of respiratory and ear infections and are more likely to develop asthma, bronchitis, and pneumonia

    7.   infants of smokers have a four times greater risk of dying of SIDS

I.   Secondhand smoke or environmental tobacco smoke (ETS)

    1.   In 1993, the EPA declared ETS a carcinogen and estimated 3,000 American nonsmokers die each year from lung cancer caused by breathing the smoke of other people's cigarettes.

    2.   comes from two sources

      a.   mainstream smoke exhaled by the smoker

      b.   sidestream smoke comes directly from a burning cigarette.

        (1)   85 percent of smoke in a room is sidestream smoke

        (2)   sidestream smoke has a two to three times higher concentration of many chemicals including nicotine, tar, and the carcinogen benzopyrene, than does mainstream smoke

J.   Quitting
1.   In 1994 , 69 percent of smokers said they would like to quit completely.
2.   nicotine is difficult to give up because when nicotine levels drop a person will experience withdrawal symptoms like severe cravings, nausea, insomnia, confusions, tremors, fatigue, headache, muscle spasms, irritability, anger, and depression
3.   forty million people have succeeded in stopping smoking.
    a.   the most successful quitters are those who do it on their own.
    b.   treatment programs have a low rate of success; 75 % of the 60 to 80 percent of those who use a cessation treatment program begin smoking again within a year
        (1)   the low success rate may be because the program provides a crutch as opposed to complete personal resolve.
    c.   replacement therapy is a method of quitting in which nicotine is provided through a patch or gum rather than obtained through a tobacco product
    d.   additional assistance may be found in support groups, acupuncture, hypnotherapy, and behavior modification therapy

K.   Benefits of quitting
1.   the body has a chance to rid itself of some of the toxins
    a.   nicotine is actually gone from the body in two to three days; respiratory passages clear
    b.   in a few days food will begin to taste and smell better
    c.   the lungs will begin to generate new tissue and you will begin to breathe easier
2.   the Surgeon General's Report in 1990 reported that people who quit smoking, regardless of their age, live longer than those who continue to smoke
3.   ten years without tobacco restores you to the same risk level as a nonsmoker

XI.   Drugs: The Use and Abuse
A.   Cannabis drugs are derived from the Cannabis sativa or Indian hemp plant and make up the Cannabis drug category.
1.   Marijuana, is the most widely used illegal drug in the United States.
    a.   approximately 10 million Americans use marijuana each month
    b.   is inexpensive, fairly simple to grow, and easy to obtain on the illicit market
2.   short term effects
    a.   disruption of short-term memory; interference with learning, reading comprehension, speech, and problem-solving abilities; difficult concentration and periods of confusion.
    b.   the drug can slow down reaction time, decrease coordination and interfere with the ability to track moving objects.
3.   long-term effects
    a.   serious studies of marijuana began over thirty years ago; the medical community warns that some negative effects may take more than thirty years to appear
    b.   there is evidence that frequent use of marijuana can lead to serious health problems, such as lung tissue damage, same respiratory problems as smokers, symptoms of chronic bronchitis and more frequent chest colds.
    c.   It takes about a month to rid the body of THC after just one use of the drug.

B. Stimulants are a group of drugs that excite the central nervous system, which means they increase heart rate, blood pressure, body temperature. Short term effects are extra energy and feeling of pleasure. The long term effects are nervousness, confusion, anxiety, loss of appetite, weight loss, malnutrition, insomnia, circulatory problems, heart complications, and strokes.

1. Cocaine is the second most popular illegal drug in the United States.
   a. in 1994, nearly 22 million Americans age twelve and older had tried cocaine at least once
   b. harvested from the leaves of the coca plant
   c. resembles flour, a fine, white, fluffy, odorless powder with a bitter taste
   d. absorbed through the nasal membranes, travels into the bloodstream, and hits the brain in about three minutes
      (1) crack is ninety percent pure cocaine and about five times as potent as street cocaine.
         (a) when smoked it takes four to six seconds to hit.
         (b) intense rush with an awful depression between hits
         (c) users will generally continue to smoke until they are out of the drug, out of money or their bodies give out.
      (2) cocaine users usually develop a congested, inflamed, constantly running nose and eventually perforate the nasal septum
      (3) a cocaine psychosis marked by paranoia and hallucinations may develop

2. Amphetamines are synthetic chemicals that are strong central nervous system stimulants.
   a. many amphetamine capsules look like their street names.
   b. can be taken as a capsules, tablets, or injections, or as powders inhaled through the nose
   c. users feel anxious, nervous, uneasy, or restless
   d. amphetamine psychosis is characterized by hallucinations, delusions, and paranoia.

3. Methamphetamine is a subgroup of amphetamines that have grown rapidly in street popularity.
   a. crank is a commonly sold methamphetamine.
      (1) ice or crystal meth is a crystallized form of crank.
         (a) more addictive than crack
         (b) easy to make.

4. Caffeine is considered a drug because high doses can result in dependency, tolerance, and withdrawal symptoms.
   a. long term heavy abuse may be linked to an increased risk of cancer, heart disease, digestive problems, and possibly pancreatic cancer
   b. fetal growth may be retarded when caffeine is abused
   c. caffeine increases alertness, which enhances attention and endurance and it suppresses appetite
   d. caffeine comes from the seeds of the coffee, cocoa and cola plants and from the leaves of the sinensis plant
      (1) may be taken in a tablet form or drunk in a beverage

    e. normal daily consumption is considered two six ounce cups of coffee, or twenty ounces of soda.

C. Hallucinogens interfere with brain chemistry by blocking or enhancing the transmission of neural signal.
  1. may block, weaken, or distort the transmission of one kind of message and enhance the transmission of another, making it stronger than it should be.
  2. most increase heart rate and blood pressure, dilate eyes, cause tremors, reduce appetite, and interfere with sleep
  3. heavy use interferes with abstract reasoning, memory and attention span
  4. two kinds of hallucinogens
    a. natural ones, found in plants; two most common:
     (1) mescaline (crown of peyote plant)
     (2) psilocybin (mushrooms)
    b. synthetic ones, which are manufactured in a laboratory, two most common:
     (1) LSD (lysergic acid diethylamide)which is 100 times stronger than psilocybin and 4,000 times stronger than mescaline
     (2) PCP (phencyclidine) a white powder, once used as a sedative by veterinarians
      (a) can be swallowed, snorted, injected, sprinkled on marijuana cigarettes and smoked, taken in liquid form, added to cocaine
      (b) decreases inhibition and provides a sense of euphoria
      (c) small doses can result in extremely violent and unpredictable behavior

D. Depressants
  1. Barbiturates
    a. synthetic drugs with short, medium, or long-lasting effects.
    b. some have important medical roles as anticonvulsants, to aid in anesthesia, and help short-term insomnia
    c. psychological addiction can occur in as little as three weeks
  2. barbiturates are generally taken by capsule or pill, but they may be injected.
  3. withdrawal symptoms include insomnia, convulsions, shaking, delirium, and hallucinations.

E. Tranquilizers
  1. are categorized as major or minor.
    a. major tranquilizers (phenothiazines) are prescribed by doctors to treat severe mental disorders.
    b. minor tranquilizers (benzodiazepines) are used to treat anxiety, insomnia, and epilepsy.
  2. in a 1990, NIDA Household survey, nearly 8.6 million Americans age twelve or older misused tranquilizers at least once

F. Opiates and Narcotics
  1. true opiate drugs are derived from the poppy plant, but in common usage the word opiate includes chemically similar synthetic drugs like methadone
    a. opium is harvested from the pods of the poppy plant and refined to become heroine, morphine, and codeine
  2. excellent painkillers with some actions that mimic endorphins

3.   in low doses or a short period of time they are not addictive, but at high doses addiction can occur in as little as two weeks of regular use

4.   usually taken in pill form and either swallowed or ground into a powder and sniffed or mixed with water, heated and then injected

5.   Heroin is highly addictive and the user must have some every eight to twelve hours or experience withdrawal symptoms of chills, nausea, aches, diarrhea, and muscle spasms.

       a.   withdrawal usually lasts three to five days, but some symptoms may linger for weeks

       b.   children may also be addicted and have to suffer withdrawal symptoms of vomiting, restlessness and seizures, which can last for several weeks

6.   Methadone is a synthetic opium which provides relief from withdrawal symptoms but is not euphoric and is therefore used in the treatment of heroin addicts

G.   Inhalants

     1.   vapors of certain legal substances can be deeply inhaled (huffed) in order to obtain a mind-altering effect

     2.   long term use can cause brain damage, hepatitis, kidney damage, violent behavior, disorientation, unconsciousness, asphyxiation, and death

H.   Designer drugs

     1.   underground chemists alter the formulas of illegal drugs enough to produce an analog, something that has roughly the same effects but is not "officially" restricted

       a.   the unpredictability of these drugs make them particularly dangerous.

       b.   analogs may be hundreds of times stronger than the original drug or have unexpected side effects

I.   Over the counter and prescription drugs

     1.   health problems from medications can be the results of taking a combination of drugs without consulting a doctor, taking the wrong amount of a drug, taking a drug more frequently than is recommended, or taking the drug for a purpose other than what was intended

     2.   prescription drugs need to be taken in the right dosage for a designated amount of time or else the medicine may be rendered ineffective and complications may result

J.   Treatment for drug-related problems

     1.   treatment programs are often tailored to specific addictions; some are tailored to meet specific cultural, gender, and sexual orientations

     2.   two basic types of programs

       a.   outpatient treatment

          (1)   drop-in center

          (2)   structured counseling and therapy program

       b.   residential treatment

          (1)   require patients to live in a controlled environment during detoxification and counseling

          (2)   work on problem and causative factors away from pressures of the "real" world

          (3)   outpatient counseling or group home living generally follow residential treatment programs

XII. Abuse Prevention: Reaching Out
   A. People trying to overcome addictions or bad habits need support.
   B. Friends and family are the most likely to spot a problem early.
   C. It is important to be informed when trying to help someone with a drug problem.
   D. Acts of prevention include helping young people get involved in healthy activities.

BEHAVIOR BOOSTS: STAGE-BASED STUDENT ACTIVITIES

For Alcohol

Precontemplator
- With the help of a friend think back over the last month and count the number of times you
   - Became sick from drinking
   - Said or did something while intoxicated that you regretted later.
   - Had alcohol-induced blackout spells or memory losses.
   - Drove home under the influence, or didn't remember how you got home.
   - Had a fight with a friend or lover while intoxicated.
   - Had a friend or family member express concern about your drinking habits.
   - Asked someone to cover for you because of drinking.
- Keep track of how much money you spend in a typical week and then figure out what percent is being spent on alcohol.
- Stop and ask yourself, Right now, where do I have alcohol?
   - In a cupboard
   - In my vest pocket or purse.
   - In the car.
   - In a drawer at work.
   - Other.
- Look at the warning signs for drugs and alcohol and circle any items that are true about you. Have a friend do the same thing about you and compare your lists.
- Watch a television show, or movie, or visit an Alcoholics Anonymous meeting to learn about alcohol abuse and its effect on the abuser and on the abuser's family and friends.

Contemplator
- Call a hotline and talk to someone about how you are considering changing. The people there can supply a friendly anonymous ear and also give you the names and phone numbers of help services.
- Talk to a recovering alcoholic.
- Think of some things you can do instead of drinking when you get the urge to drink.
- Make a list of reasons why you are thinking of cutting down or quitting drinking alcohol.
- Gather information on alcohol abuse and addiction.
- Think about who you could ask to help you overcome alcohol abuse, for example, a friend, member of the family, clergy member or other professional.

Preparer
- Tell the people you've always asked to cover for you to stop, and ask for their support in making a change.

- Try to identify what caused you to start abusing alcohol.
  - Deepening crisis in life.
  - Loneliness.
  - Academic pressure.
  - Social freedom
- Find out about help organizations like Alcoholics Anonymous (AA). Find out when they meet, and where. Check on-campus resources—counselors and services are available on every campus.
- For two weeks write down where you were, who you were with, and what you were doing when you were drinking.
- Every time you have a drink, drink it out of the same glass.
- Try to substitute drinking activities such as going to a bar with non-alcohol-related activities like miniature golf or a movie.

Action Taker
- Avoid salty foods when drinking; bars often provide them to keep you thirsty.
- Always measure the alcohol, don't just pour it into a glass.
- Eat first. This leaves less time to drink and slows alcohol absorption.
- Decline a drink you don't want.
- Offer to be the designated driver. Use this opportunity to observe the changes alcohol makes in your companions.
- Eat your money rather than drink it—order hors d'oeuvres or a sandwich instead of a drink.
- If you are thirsty, drink water or a soda first. This will keep you from gulping down an alcoholic drink.
- Choose your social settings wisely—it's easy to abstain if you go to a mall, roller blading or a movie instead of to a bar.
- Make a pact with a friend or relative that you can call for a ride anytime—no questions asked. This agreement can be used to avoid driving under the influence, but also as a way of getting out of a situation that is tempting you to drink more than you want to.
- Drink at a place where you know you can walk home or get a safe ride.
- Dilute your drink with extra fruit juice, water, soda, or ice.
- Carry a fake drink such as ginger ale with lime.
- Put the glass down between sips.
- Select and regularly attend a support group meeting like AA.
- Check into a treatment program.
-

Maintainer
- Make a plan for how you will handle a stressful situation or crisis without reaching for alcohol.
- Either avoid situations in which you would be tempted to abuse alcohol, or make a plan for how to handle such situations.
- Become the designated driver so that you have social support for not drinking.
- Ask others not to bring you alcohol as a favor.
- Celebrate achievements and holidays by doing something fun that doesn't involve alcohol, such as renting a boat, taking a day trip, golfing, sending a good friend a ticket to visit you, or treating yourself to an hour with a personal trainer at your favorite gym.
- As needed, continue to attend support group meetings.

For Tobacco

Precontemplator

- Make a list of the people you know who have died from, or are presently sick as a result of tobacco-related illness.
- Read a pamphlet describing the dangers of secondhand smoke and tobacco-related diseases.
- If you agree that secondhand smoke is a health threat, how do you feel about you, or another smoker, exposing other people, especially children, to its harmful effects?
- Visit someone who is sick with lung cancer or other tobacco-related disease.
- Make a mental note of any time that you find smoking or chewing tobacco interrupts what you are doing.
- Consider whether you would encourage or discourage a nonsmoking friend to start smoking. Your 18-year-old daughter or son?

Contemplator

- Gather information on how to quit smoking or stop using other tobacco products by visiting your doctor's office, student health clinic, or library.
- Make a list of all the reasons why you want to quit and post it in a highly visible location.
- Talk with someone who has quit smoking or chewing recently and also with someone who quit over six months ago.
- Think about how you feel about other people's smoke. Does it bother you?
- Take notice of how other people react to you when you smoke or chew or when they find out you use tobacco products. Does it affect your employment? Dating? Family life? Does the reaction of others bother you?
- Keep track of the money you spend on tobacco products. Include related expenses also, such as additional dry cleaning.
- Think about who you could depend upon to help you quit. Also consider who might make it difficult and how you could limit that influence.
- Think about what method of quitting you would try. For example, going cold turkey, joining a support group, using a nicotine replacement product.

Preparer

- Set a date to quit and post it somewhere where you will see it every day, or tell people who will support you in your effort when you are planning to quit.
- Jot down when you feel the urge to smoke or chew and the circumstances surrounding it. Also note how much time passes between cravings.
- Have your teeth cleaned and your clothing dry-cleaned before the date on which you plan to quit.
- Sign up for a smoking cessation course.
- Look for someone else who wants to quit and plan to do it together. Or look for a friend who is a reformed smoker or a nonsmoker who will help you.
- Buy cigarettes by the pack instead of by the carton.
- Delay your first cigarette or chew of the day for twenty minutes.
- Use one ashtray and wash it between uses. If you chew, spit into only one container. The idea is to make these habits inconvenient.
- Collect all your cigarette butts in one place.

- Smoke with your opposite hand or place smokeless tobacco in your mouth using your opposite hand. This will make you more aware of what you are doing.
- Do things that make it physically difficult to smoke, such as taking a shower, going for a run, swim or bike ride.
- Try quitting for increasingly long times. Quit for an hour, then half a day, one day, and so forth, until you've kicked the habit.
- Cut down on the number of cigarettes or the amount of smokeless tobacco you use every day.

Action Taker
- Don't carry cigarettes or other forms of tobacco.
- Throw away all your tobacco products and ashtrays.
- Sit in the nonsmoking sections of restaurants and other public places.
- Take a cessation course.
- Look yourself in the mirror every morning and say, "I can do it."
- Reward yourself at predetermined intervals for being tobacco free. Rewards might include new clothing, a long-distance phone call to a friend, or tickets to a game.
- Make rules about the use of tobacco in your living space. If someone starts smoking near you in a public place where smoking is permitted, move. If someone starts smoking in a nonsmoking area, politely ask them to stop.
- Make plans of action for tempting situations. Include friends who can help you. For example, if your craving for tobacco becomes too great during a social occasion ask a friend to leave with you. You can always return later when you feel in control.

Maintainer
- Avoid places or situations that would tempt you to use tobacco products, or have a plan for what you will do in these situations if you are tempted.
- Remove all tobacco products from your residence, car, knapsack or briefcase, and workplace.
- Maintain "house rules" that prohibit others from using tobacco products in your living place and car.
- Establish plans of action for how to handle tempting situations like the following examples:
    A date you didn't know smokes pulls out a pack of cigarettes or some smokeless tobacco.
    It is time to go home for the holidays with relatives who smoke or use other tobacco products.
    A client or your boss smokes during a business meeting.
- Develop new habits such as exercise that are healthy and difficult to combine with tobacco use.
- Reinforce your commitment to not smoking or using other tobacco products by helping someone else quit.
- Encourage restaurants in your area to become non-smoking establishments.

For Drug Abuse

Precontemplator
- Keep track of the money you are spending on drugs.
- Find out the legal penalty for use of an illegal substance.
- Look at your friends who do drugs and those who don't. Do you see any differences in terms of grades, financial difficulties or personality traits?
- Ask some friends whose opinions you value whether they think you have a drug problem.
- Get a physical examination.

Contemplator
- Talk with a recovering addict, either someone you know, or someone you contact through a drug hotline or other organization.
- Find out where you can get help if you decide you want it. Carry the phone number with you at all times.
- Gather information concerning the drug you think you are abusing by visiting your doctor's office, student health clinic, or library.
- Make a list of all the reasons why you want to quit and post it in a highly visible location.
- Think about how you would feel drug free.
- Take notice of how other people react to you when you use a drug or when someone finds out you use a drug. Does it affect your employment? Dating? Family life? Do other people's reactions bother you?
- Keep track of the money you spend on drugs. Include related expenses such as missed work days, destruction of property.
- Think about who you could depend on to help you quit. Also consider who might make it difficult and how you could limit that influence.
- Think about what method of quitting you would try. Examples include: cold turkey, counseling, support groups, and outpatient or inpatient treatment programs.

Preparer
- Use one of the awareness strategies (for example: smoking with your opposite hand) to make yourself aware of how often and how much you smoke.
- Decide what you would do first if you decided to quit.
- Set a date to quit and post it where you will see it every day, or tell people who will support you in your effort when you are planning to quit.
- Do not share needles (or other works) with someone else. If you must reuse equipment, clean it with bleach three times.
- If you think you will be tempted to use drugs that will influence your ability to drive, give your keys to someone you know will remain drug free.
- Jot down when you feel the urge to use a drug and the circumstances surrounding it. Also note how much time passes between cravings.
- Sign up for a treatment program.
- Look for someone else who wants to quit and plan to do it together. Or look for a friend who is drug free who will help you.
- Do things that make it physically difficult to use drugs, such as going on a long hike without taking any drugs along.

Action Taker
- Avoid putting yourself in a social situation where substances are likely to be abused, or where you feel others may try to pressure you to participate in the use of substances that are unhealthy.
- Throw away all drugs, dealer's phone numbers, and so forth. Do not carry a pager or cellular phone.
- Participate in a treatment program or support group.
- Look yourself in the mirror every morning and say "I can do it."
- Reward yourself for being drug free at pre-determined intervals. Rewards might include new clothing, a long-distance phone call to a friend, tickets to game.

- Make rules about the use of drugs in your living space. If someone offers drugs to you in your home, ask the person to leave. If the person won't leave, be prepared to follow up with a telephone call to the police. If drugs are offered to you somewhere else, leave immediately and call a supportive friend.
- Make plans of actions for tempting situations. Include friends who can help you. For example, carry the phone number of a supportive person and a hotline that is available twenty-four hours a day.

Maintainer
- Do not ride in a car with someone who is under the influence of any type of drug, or in possession of illegal drugs.
- Surround yourself with friends who don't abuse drugs.
- Avoid places or situations that would tempt you to use drugs or have a plan for what you will do in these situations if you are tempted.
- remove all drug products and paraphernalia from your residence, car, knapsack or briefcase, and workplace.
- Maintain "house rules" that prohibit others from using drugs in your living place and car.
- Establish plans of action for how to handle tempting situations like the following examples:
    A date offering you a drug.
    A dealer pushing you to buy.
    Free drugs at a party.
- Reinforce your commitment to not using drugs by helping someone else quit.
- Become involved in a community effort to stop the abuse of drugs, such as a school education program, a neighborhood watch, or a peer counseling program.

For Abuse Prevention

Precontemplator
- Think about how you would feel if a relative or good friend were killed by a drunk driver. Would you wish someone had stopped the drunk driver from getting into the car? Have you ever watched an intoxicated person or someone under the influence of drugs leave with car keys?
- Think of a situation where someone did something for you that saved you from embarrassment, harm, or injury. Would you like to be that type of person?
- Think about how you feel when you hear about drug-addicted babies and children with fetal alcohol syndrome. Do you wish that you could do something to prevent children from being innocent victims?
- Have you ever been one of a crowd of people who did not respond to someone's needs or cries of help, and later wished that you had?

Contemplator
- Role play how you would like to respond in different situations. Examples: What would you say to an intoxicated friend who is about to get in the car and drive? What you would do if you saw someone you know (or don't know) buying drugs or sharing needles?
- Ask someone who is involved in community service about what they do and why they do it. Visit your campus financial aid office and ask about community service work opportunities.
- Choose a cause (such as MADD, DARE, Big Sister, or Big Brother program) and call, visit or write for additional information on volunteer opportunities.
- Talk among your friends and see if they are interested in volunteering as a group for projects such as Habitat for Humanity.

- Find out how to become a substance abuse peer counselor by visiting the student health clinic, student development office or student counseling center.

Preparer

- Role play how you would handle situations that involve substance abuse, then make a commitment that the next time you are in such a situation you will take action.
- Attend several meetings and join one organization such as MADD or DARE if you like what you see and hear.
- Spend one evening at a hotline center to see if it is something you would be interested in doing.
- Write or call for informational materials on one form of substance abuse, and obtain permission to post promotional material on campus bulletin boards. (Or volunteer to help the health and counseling offices get the word out on campus.)
- Approach a friend and offer assistance. (Be prepared for anger and denial.)
- Make a decision on how much time you can commit to community involvement, and then select an activity that will fit in the time period you have determined. There are positive actions that take as little as ten minutes (for example, calling a cab or giving someone a ride home) and others that require major time commitments (for example, peer counseling).
- Experiment with some of the other activities listed under Action Taker.

Action Taker

- Support preventive education, reinforce the ideas that young people are learning. Ask children what they've learned about substance abuse in school. Then role play refusal skills with them.
- Be a role model. People often wait to see what members of a group to do, and then they join in. Don't be afraid to say no to drugs, or to another drink. Your behavior will encourage others in the group to make wise choices. When discussing college life with young people, be sure to talk about your classes and activities, rather than just talking about how great the parties are.
- Be a hotline volunteer.
- Be a designated driver. Take the keys away from a friend who is intoxicated. Prevent others from driving drunk by alerting the manager of a restaurant/bar or alerting the police.
- Call for help when you think someone is in danger of alcohol poisoning or an overdose.
- Set rules about substance abuse in your home, dorm room, car, or presence.
- Volunteer to become a friend for a high-risk child or one who comes from a household where substance abuse occurs. You can make a difference just by exchanging letters.
- Talk to someone you care about who you think has a substance abuse problem.
- Give or anonymously mail someone an informational pamphlet or hotline number if you are worried about him or her.
- Call the police when you see a drug deal or someone driving drunk. You don't have to give your name if it will put you in danger.
- If you are an employer, set up a program to help employees and encourage self-disclosure.
- Invite someone to do something with you, such as going for a walk or playing a game of chess when you know he or she is trying to kick a habit.
- Be the one who calls for medical assistance or takes someone to the hospital when you think the person is in trouble. Don't wait to be sure—in cases of drug overdose and alcohol poisoning, the sooner treatment is begun the better.
- Put up posters or bumper stickers that encourage drug-free activity or that advertise where help is available.

- Call one of the many support groups and see if they need volunteer help. Even if you don't have a lot of time, they may have onetime jobs like helping to fold pamphlets.
- Become a part of an alternative program for people of all ages. Communities need volunteers to run youth organizations and athletic programs. Loneliness can lead to substance abuse. Think about people who live alone and invite them to join you for a meal or other activity; you don't have to wait for a holiday.
- Volunteer to help run a campus health fair or awareness week activity.
- Help an intoxicated stranger get home safely by calling a cab or bringing the problem to the attention of the management.
- If you have been enabling someone to continue a bad habit by covering for him or her, stop.
- Stop serving or drinking alcoholic beverages an hour before the end of a party or function.
- When throwing a party offer plenty of nonalcoholic beverages. For example, you might tap a keg of root beer.
- If you see unusual driving habits, back off or take a turn to get away from the car, and report the license plate and make of the car to the police as soon as possible.
- Walk an intoxicated friend home.

Maintainer
- Limit your involvement so that it does not overtax your ability to keep up with your studies and other commitments.
- Keep a fresh perspective on involvement by trying a new activity.
- Invite friends to volunteer with you. If you have a friend involved with an organization, join in.
- Work together with others when confronting a friend or family member with a substance abuse problem.

ADDITIONAL STUDENT ACTIVITIES

Activity 14.1 Helping or Hurting (page 318) An activity to identify enabling behaviors.
Activity 14.2 Why Do You Smoke (page 324)

LABS

Lab 14.1 What Can I Do? (pages 341–344)
Lab 14.2 Do You Have A Problem With Alcohol? (page 345)
Lab 14.3 Drug Awareness (page 346)

RESOURCES

Suggested Reading

Alcoholics Anonymous, 3rd ed. New York: Alcoholics Anonymous World Services, 1976.

Avis, H. *Drugs and life*. Dubuque, IA: Brown & Benchmark, 1990.

Blum, K. *Alcohol and the addictive brain: New hope for alcoholics from biogenetic research.* New York: Fress Press, 1991.

Cocores, J. *The 800-COCAINE book of drug and alcohol recovery.* New York: Villard Books, 1990.

Dorris, M. *The broken cord.* New York: Harper-Collins, 1992.

Gibbons, B. The preventable tragedy-fetal alcohol syndrome. *National Geographic* 181(2), February, 1992.

Hermes, W.J. *Substance abuse (The encyclopedia of health),* New York: Chelsea House Publishers, 1993.

Nakken, C. *The addictive personality: Understanding compulsion in our lives.* Hazelton Foundation, Center City, NM. New York: Harper & Row Publishers, 1988.

Schlaadt, R. *Drugs, society and behavior.* Guildford, CT: Dushkin Publishing Company, 1992.

U.S. Department of Heath and Human Services. *Healthy people 2000: National health promotion and disease prevention objectives.* DHHS Publication No. (PHS) 91-50214. Washington, D.C.: U. S. Government Printing Office, 1990.

Organizations

Action on Smoking and Health
2013 4th Street, NW
Washington, DC 20006
Tel: (202) 659-4310
Web site: http://www.ash.org

Alcohol and Drug Problems Association of North America
444 N. Capital Street, NW, Suite 706
Washington, DC 20001

Alcoholic Anonymous
AA World Services, Inc.
P.O. Box 459, Grand Central Station
New York, NY 10163
Tel: (212) 870-3400
Web site: http://www.alcohols-anonymous.org

American Council on Alcohol Problems
3426 Bridgeland Drive
Bridgeton, MO 63044

American Council for Drug Education
204 Monroe Street
Rockville, MD 20850
Web site: http://www.acde.org

Alcohol Research Information Service
1106 E. Oakland
Lansing, MI 48906
Web site: http://www.silk.nih.gov/silk/niaa/others/resources
American Heart Association
National Center
7272 Greenville Avenue
Dallas, TX 75231
Tel (800) AHA-USA1 (Customer Heart & Stroke Information)
Tel (888) MY-HEART (Women's Health Information)
Web site: http://www.aha.org

Breathe-Free Plan to Stop Smoking
6830 Laurel Street, NW
Washington, DC 20012

Center for Substance Abuse Prevention (CSAP)
(301) 443-0373

Infoline
(800) 203-1234

Mothers Against Drunk Drivers (MADD)
(800) 544-3690

National Clearinghouse for Alcohol and Drug
Information (NCADI)
P.O. Box 2345
Rockville, MD 20847-2345
Tel: (800) 729-6686
Web site: http://health.org

National Council on Alcoholism and Drug
Dependence
(800) 622-6255

National Institute on Alcohol and Alcoholism
Web site: http://www.niaaa.nih.gov

National Interagency Council on Smoking and
Health
c/o American Heart Association
7320 Greenville Avenue
Dallas, TX 75231
Tel (800) AHA-USA1 (Customer Heart & Stroke
Information)
Tel (888) MY-HEART (Women's Health
Information)
Web site: http://www.aha.org

Smokenders
666 11th Street, NW
Washington, DC 20001
Tel: (800) 828-4357
Web site: http://smokenders.com

Tobacco Control Resources
Tobacco Control Groups and addresses
Boston, MA
Web site:
http://www.tobacco.org/resources/tob_adds

Video
The Drug Tape. Realistic dramatization. Effects of
various drugs. No nonsense approach. Cambridge.

Additional Local and Community Resources
Alcoholism Foundation
Blue Cross/Blue Shield
Drug Counseling services (local or state mental
health facilities)
Social Services agencies (state or private)
State Department of Health
State Division of Alcohol and Drugs

Living Well in Today's World

Chapter 15

CHAPTER SUMMARY

You are ultimately responsible for your own behavior and in control of your lifestyle habits; however, you should recognize that your actions will be influenced by both your human-cultural and natural environments. These influences can be very positive and supportive, or they can make change difficult. Try to find ways to meld personal desires with those of people around you. This helps foster positive relationships and a healthy society. Sometimes, however, you may be faced with a destructive or hostile environment that threatens your efforts to make or sustain healthy choices. In these instances, you may have to leave the environment (such as an abusive home) or seek an intervention (such as counseling) in order to change your environment or change how you react to it. In many cases, however, a negative environment can be turned into a supportive one through communication, compromise, and positive example. Furthermore, open yourself to the possibility that you can do more to enrich, and less to harm the environment, and look for proactive ways to accomplish this. Like the ripples of a stone tossed into a pond, the positive changes you make will touch all life around you.

LEARNING OBJECTIVES

The student will be able to:
- develop strategies for making long-term behavior changes.
- articulate why relapse is common when making change, and identify triggers for relapse.
- explain the relationship between the stages of change and relapse.
- explain how quality of life requires respect for, and is influenced by, the environment.
- explain what it means to make personal wellness decisions within the context of world wellness.
- identify positive and negative ways that the human-cultural environment affects lifestyle choices.
- identify positive and negative ways that personal lifestyle choices affect the human-cultural environment.
- identify positive and negative ways that the natural environment affects lifestyle choices.
- identify positive and negative ways that personal lifestyle choices affect the natural environment.

PERSONAL PROFILE

You—The Student

No personal profile is provided. Instead, students are encouraged to profile themselves or someone like a friend, mentor, or family member who exemplifies a wellness lifestyle in a way that reflects consideration for the human-cultural and natural environments. Or a profile can be about the way the student or someone else handled relapse and was able to move ahead with a lifestyle change.

CONTENT OUTLINE

I. Wellness is a lifetime committed to healthy behaviors.
   A. An illness/treatment approach is a short-term fix to a long-term problem.
   B. Responsible personal wellness includes making behavior decisions with consideration for other people and the natural environment.

II. Change
   A. The process can be both exciting and scary, especially in the beginning.
   B. Creates good and bad stress and some people avoid change to avoid stress.
   C. Requires time, effort, and patience.
   D. Is most successful when taken one step at a time using strategies that match a person's readiness to change (precontemplator, contemplator, preparer, action taker, maintainer).
   E. With time new behaviors become more comfortable than old behaviors.
   F. The environment often changes when a person maintains a new behavior—usually in a way that supports the new behavior (e.g., a person who quits smoking may make new friends who don't smoke or inspire old friends to quit too.)

III. Relapse
   A. Is a natural part of the process of change
   B. When unexpected or stressful events arise, it is easy to revert back to old behaviors.
   C. Regression can happen at any stage from contemplator to maintainer.
   D. Think of relapse not as failure but as a temporary detour on the road of success.
   E. Avoid disliking yourself for relapse.
   F. Make a plan ahead of time as to how you will get going again if you relapse.
   G. The longer you maintain a new behavior the more comfortable it becomes and the less likely you are to relapse.

IV. World Wellness
   A. A world view recognizes that there is an interconnectedness between ourselves and our environment (people, places, animals, plants, etc.).
      1. human beings are part of a larger ecosystem
      2. our behavior affects the people and environment around us
      3. the people and environment around us affect our behavior
   B. Personal lifestyle decisions are best made within the greater context of world wellness.

V. The Human-Cultural Environment
   A. Made up of the people who surround us, plus their laws, religious beliefs, traditions, and social mores

B. As the ability to communicate around the world "shrinks" the world, the whole human race becomes our human cultural environment but for change usually those closest to us have the most influence.
  1. human cultural environments are defined by these and other characteristics:
     a. ethnicity
     b. religion
     c. geographic location
     d. sexual preference
     e. economic prosperity
  2. local human cultural environments can be very different
     a. retirement community vs. mixed age neighborhood
     b. single race suburb vs. a mixed race suburb vs. a race specific urban neighborhood

C. The human cultural environment influences the individual's wellness behaviors and decisions.
  1. values are learned from parents, relatives, friends, neighbors, teachers, and spiritual leaders
  2. traditions are taught from birth to adulthood and passed from one generation to the next
  3. language and culture shape thinking and actions
  4. people from different human cultural environments may approach decisions from different frames of reference
  5. to become more aware of your own culture, experience a different one
     a. travel abroad
     b. talk with a foreign student
     c. visit a different church or temple
     d. attend ethnic festivals
     e. take a course in comparative religions, human diversity, world history
  6. college life may place you in a new and different human cultural environment
  7. the human-cultural environment can have both a positive and negative influence
     a. belonging: family or gang
     b. work: challenge or stress
     c. peers: friendship or peer pressure to drink, use drugs, etc.
  8. lifestyle changes are easiest when the change aligns with your human-cultural environment because you receive support for your efforts
  9. it is difficult to make lifestyle changes when they disagree with the beliefs or practices of the human-cultural environment
     a. for example it is harder to abstain from premarital sex when peers are encouraging it, society condones it, and the media "advertises it"
     b. in some cases, complete removal from the present human-cultural environment is needed (e.g., checking into a drug rehabilitation center)
  10. technological advancements have influenced lifestyle
     a. positive influence examples:
        (1) more leisure time
        (2) less physical stress
        (3) more done in less time
     b. negative influence examples

          (1)   added work/psychological stress by making things happen faster and allowing a person to be available to work 24 hours a day (fax, cell phone, etc.)

          (2)   new health concerns like carpal tunnel syndrome

          (3)   more sedentary life

D.   Each of us influences our human-cultural environment.

    1.   as we strive to improve personal wellness, it is important to be aware of, and responsible for, the impact of our actions on other people, on our culture, on our heritage, and on the rules of society

    2.   positive examples:

        a.   one person making a positive change often influences others to do likewise

        b.   safe sex protects self and partner from disease and unwanted pregnancy

        c.   healthy cooking improves the diet of all who eat with you

    3.   negative examples:

        a.   smoking results in others inhaling second-hand smoke

        b.   drug and alcohol abuse can result in abusive behavior toward others

        c.   poor stress management can result in tension between self and others

E.   Making change usually affects other people.

    1.   one person's change may motivates others to do likewise

    2.   one person's change may embarrass someone unwilling to change, in which case that person may bad mouth the other person's attempt to change

        a.   treat as a precontemplator and try to help raise the person's awareness

    3.   one person's change may disrupt others

        a.   as an example, roller blading is good physical activity with health benefits but skaters can be a problem to pedestrians and traffic

        b.   look for solutions that result in win-win situations such as marking routes for roller bladers or creating a roller blading area

    4.   sometimes healthy changes are in conflict with present traditions/ideas for example:

        a.   some cultures do not encourage women to be physically active

        b.   promoting anti-smoking measures is more difficult when income comes from tobacco crops

F.   Gathering support for your decision to change

    1.   educate others, explain why you are adopting a new lifestyle habit

    2.   ask others to join you, some changes are easier to do with a partner or a group

    3.   look for win-win solutions when your change disrupts others

    4.   allow others time to adjust to your decision

VI.   The natural environment: everything nonhuman

A.   Each of us influences the wellness of the natural world.

    1.   human-centered perspective

        a.   world exists to fulfill human needs

        b.   things with human uses are valuable, those that are not useful are devalued

        c.   has led to a depletion of resources and disruption of plant/animal ecosystems

    2.   shift from human-centered to world view or world ecosystem view

        a.   we don't dominate the world, rather we are stewards of it

        b.   can't just consume, must work toward sustainability

        c.   look at the consequences of actions with the "bigger picture" in mind

        d.   balance industry and profit with concern for the environment

        e.   shift from believing we have the "right" to something to having "responsibility" for the whole ecosystem

3.   many people now live somewhat removed from the natural world

        a.   technology allows us to regulate lighting, temperature, etc., so that outdoor conditions control our lives less

        b.   grocery stores remove us from the reality of growing and harvesting food

        c.   difficult to appreciate how the environment is being impacted when you are removed from it

4.   there is a need to regain awareness of the environment, its rhythms, our interconnectedness with it

        (1)   awareness can be achieved through outdoor recreation

        (2)   natural disasters re-focus attention on nature

        (3)   education can help raise awareness

B.   The natural environment's influence on us.

1.   the pattern of our lives is tied into the rhythms of our environment such as the passing seasons, rise and fall of tides, and days turning into nights

2.   the natural resources around us determine to some extent what we do for a living, what we eat, how we play

3.   the food we eat is tied into what grows in our geographic area although this is changing with the easy transportation and refrigeration of foods

        a.   traditional diets changing with new food availability has enhanced nutrition in some areas and created problems for others

        (1)   American Indians have in some cases had increased problems with obesity and diabetes with a change from their traditional diet

        b.   Americans have learned from other cultures to eat less red meat to reduce incidence of heart disease

4.   the climate and geography influence our choice of physical activities

        a.   people in warm weather climates tend to be more physically active than those living with long, cold winters

        (1)   this can be compensated for by participating in outdoor winter activities or by using an indoor recreation facility (including home exercise equipment)

        b.   heat and humidity can limit outdoor physical activity

        (1)   exercise early in the day before the heat rises

        (2)   on hot humid days switch to indoor activities or outdoor activities like swimming

        c.   pollen and air pollution, especially in urban areas, can especially restrict the activity level of those who suffer allergies and asthma

        (1)   to cut down on inhalation of car exhaust, exercise early in the morning

        (2)   check the air quality index before exercising outdoors in urban or high pollution areas

        (3)   exercise indoors on high pollen or pollution day

        d.   rain

        (1)   switch to indoor activities

        (2)   purchase rain gear and be active outside

        e.   geographic area

(1)   different areas offer different opportunities for physical activity; for example:

    (a)   rivers: boating, fishing, swimming

    (b)   mountains: hiking, skiing, mountain biking

5.   climate influences life patterns and health

    a.   schedules are set around climate: school, construction, farming, etc.

        (1)   weather can affect people's health

        (2)   long dark winters or rainy seasons can cause depression in some people

        (3)   some people love the heat, others the cold (regulated heating and cooling systems have tempered some of these problems)

        (4)   people in sunny climates tend to be more physically active but also have a higher incidence of skin cancer (preventable with sun block, etc.)

6.   stress and relaxation can both be products of the natural environment

    a.   stress examples

        (1)   noise especially in urban centers

        (2)   city person nervous in the woods; country person uptight in the city

    b.   relaxation examples

        (1)   outdoor recreation to get away from pressures of home and work

        (2)   outdoor physical activity often results in a relaxation response

        (3)   gardening, fishing, etc., are enjoyed by many

7.   the natural environment has many "looks"

    a.   there is wildlife and plant life in the city as well as the country

    b.   outdoor recreation can be hiking a trail or up a monument's stairs

    c.   a bike ride or walk can take you along city streets, small town roads, or along a river in the woods

VII.   Things the individual can do for the natural environment

    A.   Create less garbage.

    B.   Carpool or drive less.

    C.   Recycle.

    D.   Purchase recyclable products.

    E.   Avoid products that are bad for the environment

    F.   Treat wildlife in a way that lets them remain "wild."

    G.   Join or create a group that works toward the welfare of the environment.

BEHAVIOR BOOSTS: STAGE-BASED STUDENT ACTIVITIES

No specific stage-based behavior boosts are offered for this chapter although the suggested activities below range from awareness type activities to action/maintenance type activities. Behavior boosts were not developed for this chapter, as the material is more about the change process and philosophical views concerning personal and world wellness and less about specific lifestyle behaviors.

ADDITIONAL SUGGESTED STUDENT ACTIVITIES

Activity 1: Your Environment and Change

Answer the questions in Activity 15.1 (text page 349) concerning the role of the environment and your attempts to change lifestyle behaviors.

Activity 2: Whose Wellness Is Important?

Answer the questions in Activity 15.2 (text page 352) concerning how to balance one's own wellness needs with the needs of other people and the natural environment.

Activity 3: The Impact of Societal Rules and Mores on the Individual

- Societal rules, traditions, religious beliefs, and mores have an impact on every individual living within a society. Can you think of any examples of how these rules have had an impact on you? Here are a few examples to get you started:

- Illegal drug use: Laws prohibit it. Communities support a drug-free lifestyle by providing educational programs, rehabilitation programs and law enforcement. At the same time, illicit drugs are readily available, there is peer pressure to experiment, and in some situations such as gang life there is an expectation of use. How has your human-cultural environment shaped your beliefs about using drugs? Are there conflicting views among the people you know? If so, whom do you believe and why?

- Alcohol consumption: Variations across culture as to how acceptable alcohol use is and what is too much. If you profess a religion, have religious teachings influenced your use of alcohol?

- Eating: Tradition usually plays a big role. As an adult, do you eat the same kinds of foods you ate growing up? Does ethnic background play a role in what you eat?

- Getting a tan: Tanning has been shown to increase skin cancer risk. Do the people around you discourage tanning, or is a spring break tan still desirable? How do other's opinions influence your behavior?

List some of your ideas here:

Activity 4: Challenging the Norm: Individuals Can Make a Difference

The individual can positively affect the wellness of his or her human-cultural environment. Some acts influence only a small group of people, while other acts influence a nation or even the world. An individual may cause a family rule to be changed or national legislation to be rewritten. Both levels are important to the wellness of our society.

Here are just a few examples of individuals who have changed the way their human-cultural environments think:

1. Jack Kevorkian, MD, is a pathologist who developed the controversial assisted-suicide machine. He has been arrested for helping terminally ill patients end their lives, but has never been convicted. Instead states have reexamined their laws.

2. Joan Benoit is a 1988 Olympic gold medalist in the marathon. She admits that when she first started running, she would pretend to pick flowers when a car went by rather than be "seen" running. Her successful career has legitimized long distance running for women especially in the United States.

3. Maya Angelou is an African American author, poet and entertainer who has used her literary talents to focus attention on human potential. She inspired the nation with her poem, "On the Pulse of the Morning," which she read at President Clinton's 1993 inauguration.

4. Mahatma Gandhi was an Indian nationalist leader who established his country's freedom through a nonviolent revolution. Imprisoned numerous times, he effectively used fasting and passive resistance to free India from British rule. Gandhi's teaching inspired nonviolent movements elsewhere including the movement in the United States by civil rights activist Martin Luther King, Jr.

Can you think of an individual (past or present) who has had a positive (or negative) influence on society? The influence need not be as broad as the examples given.

Can you think of things you have done which have influenced the wellness of those around you?

Activity 5: You and the Natural Environment

Read the Cognitive Corner, You Can Make a Difference, on pages 354–355 in the textbook and see if there is one thing in the list you think you would like to do to help care for the natural environment.

RESOURCES

Organizations

Human Ecology Action League
P.O. Box 29629
Atlanta, GA 30359
Web site: www.snre.edu/gain/se

National Conference of Local Environmental
Health Administrators
2405 S. Liberty Street
Albany, OR 97231

National Environmental Health Association
720 S. Colorado Blvd., Suite 970, South Tower
Denver, CO 80222
Tel: (303) 756-9090
Fax: (303) 691-9490
Web site: www.csn.net

Greenpeace, USA, Inc.
1436 U Street, NW
Washington, DC 20009
Tel: (202) 462-1177
Web site: Greenpeace.usa@wdc.greenpeace.org

National Audubon Society
700 Broadway
New York, NY 10003
Tel: (212) 979-3000

National Wildlife Federation
1400 16th Street NW
Washington, DC 20036
Tel: (202) 797-4600

The Nature Company
1815 North Lynn Street
Arlington, VA 22209
Tel: (703) 841-5300

Sierra Club
730 Polk Street
San Francisco, CA 94109
Tel: (415) 776-2211

Test Bank Preface

Test questions were created using three different formats: multiple choice, true/false, and essay questions. All questions have the correct response shown directly after the questions. Following the correct responses for multiple choice questions is a number shown in parentheses. This number ranges from 1–3 and is a measure of the difficulty of the question. Questions marked with a 1 are the easiest and tend to be factual. Questions marked with a 3 are the most difficult. Mix and match questions of varying difficulty as you prepare your exams.

Multiple Choice

1. Wellness is best described as:
   a. a state of good physical fitness.
   b. the absence of disease
   c. a way of life that includes personal control and the adoption of healthy lifestyle habits
   d. a state of health achieved through regular medical check-ups and treatments

   answer: C(2)

2. Which one of the following is not one of the five dimensions of wellness?
   a. social wellness
   b. nutritional wellness
   c. spiritual wellness
   d. emotional wellness

   answer: B(1)

3. Readiness to change is LEAST likely to be influenced by:
   a. personality
   b. living and working environments
   c. family support
   d. intelligence

   answer: D(2)

4. People who practice healthy lifestyle habits are more apt to:
   a. have more friends
   b. make more money
   c. have longer, higher quality lives
   d. all of the above

   answer: C(2)

5. A poor quality of life may be described as:
   a. dysfunctional living
   b. dependence upon medical services
   c. the inability to perform daily living tasks
   d. all of the above

   answer: D(2)

6. During which of the following ages did it become clear that 75 percent of all premature deaths were preventable?
   a. age of environment
   b. age of medicine
   c. age of lifestyle
   d. age of wellness

   answer: C(2)

7. According to the wellness movement, who has primary responsibility for your health and wellness?
   a. a personal physician
   b. an athletic trainer
   c. a nutritionist
   d. you

   answer: D(2)

8. A wellness lifestyle can:
   a. increase lifespan
   b. decrease the number of dysfunctional years
   c. improve quality of life for the chronically ill
   d. all of the above

   answer: D(2)

9. Physical wellness includes all of the following EXCEPT:
   a. performing regular exercise
   b. avoiding substance abuse
   c. being creative and imaginative
   d. practicing safer sex

   answer: C(2)

10. Which of the following is MOST attributed to spiritual wellness?
    a. discovering a sense of purpose
    b. managing stress
    c. developing friendships
    d. being creative and imaginative

    answer: A(2)

11. In addition to lifestyle, wellness can be influenced by:
    a. heredity
    b. environment
    c. inadequate health care
    d. all of the above

    answer: D(1)

12. People who have decided to change but who haven't consistently practiced the new behavior are:
    a. precontemplators
    b. contemplators
    c. preparers
    d. action takers

    answer: C(2)

13. Weighing the pros and cons is a useful strategy for:
    a. contemplators
    b. preparers
    c. action takers
    d. maintainers

    answer: A(2)

14. The ability to laugh at oneself is a sign of _____ wellness.
    a. emotional
    b. mental
    c. physical
    d. social

    answer: A(2)

15. The personality trait of _____ is a predictor of heart disease.
    a. hardiness
    b. hostility
    c. workaholism
    d. all of the above

    answer: B(2)

16. The ability to think clearly and make good decisions is most indicative of _____ wellness.
    a. physical
    b. mental
    c. emotional
    d. social

    answer: B(2)

17. Which of the following two people are leaders in the field of behavior change?
    a. Freud and Jung
    b. Cooper and Blair
    c. Prochaska and DiClemente
    d. Sorenson and Simmons

    answer: C(1)

18. A person who uses marijuana and sees nothing wrong with it is a:
    a. precontemplator
    b. contemplator
    c. action taker
    d. maintainer

    answer: A(3)

19. A person who wants to lose weight, has done a diet analysis, and is putting together a diet plan is a:
    a. contemplator
    b. preparer
    c. action taker
    d. maintainer

    answer: B(3)

20. A person who has been exercising regularly for a year is a:
    a. contemplator
    b. preparer
    c. action taker
    d. maintainer

    answer: D(3)

True/False

1. Programs that assume everyone is ready to change often have low rates of success. (True)

2. People tend to be in the same stage of readiness to change for most of their wellness behaviors. (False)

3. People who exercise regularly will, on the average, live longer than those who don't. (True)

4. Not everyone is equally ready to make lifestyle changes. (True)

5. Physical wellness is the most important dimension of wellness. (False)

6. People with disabilities cannot live a wellness lifestyle. (False)

7. Ninety percent of premature deaths are preventable. (False)

8. Of the average lifespan of 64 years, approximately 12 are dysfunctional years. (True)

9. While illnesses or disabilities can negatively affect quality of life, they need not deter one from living a wellness lifestyle and achieving personal potential. (True)

10. A wellness lifestyle ensures total health. (False)

11. Many people depend on medicine to fix them, rather than practice prevention. (True)

12. If you are disease free you are healthy. (False)

13. People with low levels of fitness are more likely to die from cancer or heart disease than individuals with good or excellent levels of fitness. (True)

14. Being flexible is more important to health than being agile. (True)

15. Spiritual wellness includes coming to peace with oneself and discovering a sense of purpose. (True)

16. The ability to have positive interactions with others is a sign of mental wellness. (False)

17. Inadequate or inaccessible health care can affect wellness, especially among socioeconomically depressed populations. (True)

18. A person can be in different stages for different health behaviors. (True)

19. In the Stages of Change Model, movement from one stage to another can be linear or jump stages. (True)

20. Behavior change strategies are more effective when they are stage-based. (True)

21. Developing a plan of action usually occurs in the contemplation stage. (False)

22. Identifying supports and barriers is especially important in the early stages of change. (True)

23. Goal setting is a key strategy for the maintenance stage. (False)

Short Answer/Essay

1. Define wellness, including the dimensions of wellness.

2. Explain how the definition of health has changed and explain its relationship with wellness.

3. What does it mean to take a proactive stance toward wellness? Describe five behaviors a proactive person would adopt or maintain in pursuit of wellness.

4. List and describe the four factors responsible for all causes of death.

5. Identify five behaviors that should be included in a healthy lifestyle.

6. Describe and characterize the five stages of the behavior change model. Identify a change strategy you might use for each of the five stages.

The Fitness-Wellness Connection

Multiple Choice

1. What percentage of American adults do not achieve the recommended amount of regular physical activity?
   a. 25%
   b. 40%
   c. 60%
   d. 75%

   answer: C(1)

2. The wellness movement started to take off in the:
   a. 1960s
   b. 1970s
   c. 1980s
   d. 1990s

   answer: C(1)

3. Which of the following is NOT a health-related component of physical fitness?
   a. cardiorespiratory fitness
   b. body composition
   c. flexibility
   d. agility

   answer: D(1)

4. Which of the following is NOT an immediate response to exercise?
   a. faster heart rate
   b. greater stroke volume
   c. increased ventilations
   d. increased muscular strength

   answer: D(2)

5. Which of the following fitness components is concerned with body fat?
   a. speed
   b. body composition
   c. flexibility
   d. coordination

   answer: B(1)

6. To obtain most of the health benefits, perform moderately intense physical activity for:
   a. 30 minutes on most days
   b. 20 minutes three days a week
   c. 45 minutes three to five times a week
   d. 60 minutes twice a week

   answer: A(2)

7. Which of the following is NOT a benefit of regular exercise?
   a. less muscular fatigue during normal daily tasks
   b. improved neural transmission
   c. stress reduction
   d. enhanced aggressive tendencies

   answer: D(2)

8. A physically fit person:
   a. has an enhanced functional capacity
   b. has an elevated resting heart rate
   c. is necessarily a physically skilled individual
   d. all of the above

   answer: A(2)

9. Regular exercise increases the strength of:
   a. bones
   b. ligaments
   c. tendons
   d. all of the above

   answer: D(2)

10. Anaerobic activities usually last:
    a. 1 minute or less
    b. 3–5 minutes
    c. 6–10 minutes
    d. 20 minutes or more

    answer: A(2)

11. The physiological condition in which the consumption of oxygen meets the body's demand for oxygen is called:
    a. the "burn"
    b. interval training
    c. metabolism
    d. steady state

    answer: D(2)

12. Exercise that requires oxygen is considered:
    a. aerobic
    b. anaerobic
    c. asthmatic
    d. anabolic

    answer: A(1)

13. The "burn" does NOT :
    a. occur during intense aerobic exercise
    b. occur during intense anaerobic exercise
    c. occur when lactic acid accumulates
    d. happen as quickly to more fit individuals

    answer: A(2)

14. Which of the following statements is TRUE?
    a. Exercise induced asthma (EIA) does not respond to bronchodilator medication.
    b. Aerobic conditioning raises the exertion level at which EIA symptoms occur.
    c. People with EIA should avoid endurance exercise.
    d. Asthmatics are more apt to have an EIA attack in warm weather than cold weather.

    answer: B(2)

15. A person who wants to lose fat should use a progression of:
    a. intensity
    b. speed
    c. duration
    d. frequency

    answer: C(2)

16. The overload principle is characterized by:
    a. working to the point of pain
    b. the overuse syndrome
    c. working just beyond the usual point of tolerance
    d. detraining

    answer: C(2)

17. Progression is the gradual increase of:
    a. intensity
    b. duration
    c. frequency
    d. all of the above

    answer D(2)

18. Adding a half a mile to your walk is an example of:
    a. progressive overload
    b. specificity
    c. reversibility
    d. overuse

    answer: A(2)

19. A good warm-up would include:
    a. fast ballistic movements
    b. flexibility demanding movements
    c. slow, building to moderately paced, movements
    d. movements carefully performed with weights

    answer: C(2)

20. During the cool-down, one should:
    a. perform easy movements and static stretches
    b. perform easy movements and ballistic stretches
    c. lie down on the floor and breathe deeply
    d. perform difficult movements at a slow pace

    answer: A(2)

21. During exercise, blood flow to the:
    a. muscles increases
    b. brain decreases
    c. skin decreases
    d. stomach and kidneys increases

    answer: A(1)

22. Exercise goals should be:
    a. general and difficult to attain
    b. specific and attainable
    c. many and easy to attain
    d. few and difficult to attain

    answer: B(2)

23. Which of the following is an example of intrinsic motivation?
    a. an exercise buddy calling to make sure you are coming
    b. working toward "feeling good"
    c. betting a friend you will lose weight
    d. winning a T-shirt for regular attendance to a fitness class

    answer: B(2)

24. During exercise, blood is shunted to the:
    a. stomach
    b. active muscles
    c. intestines
    d. none of the above

    answer: B(1)

25. Factors relating to exercise adherence include:
    a. remaining free of injury
    b. attitude toward physical activity
    c. convenience of workout facility
    d. all of the above

    answer: D(1)

26. Motivation can be generated through:
    a. goal setting
    b. social approval
    c. early and on-going assessments
    d. all of the above

    answer: D(1)

27. A medical examination is recommended for all of the following EXCEPT:
    a. males over 40
    b. females over 50
    c. healthy adults under age 40
    d. those who have a chronic disease

    answer: C(1)

28. To prevent injury:
    a. develop strong muscles
    b. maintain good flexibility
    c. warm-up before being active
    d. all of the above

    answer: D(1)

True/False

1. The majority of American adults do not get enough exercise. (TRUE)

2. Recent research indicates that individuals need to exercise at higher intensities than previously thought in order to obtain most of the health benefits. (FALSE)

3. Agility is a health-related component of physical fitness. (FALSE)

4. Balance is a skill-related component of physical fitness. (TRUE)

5. Muscular strength will burn off fat. (FALSE)

6. Three 10-minute sessions of physical activity are as good as one 30-minute session. (TRUE)

7. Advanced exercisers make more dramatic increase in fitness than beginners. (FALSE)

8. Physical wellness impacts all the other dimensions of wellness. (TRUE)

9. Exercise is not recommended for people with exercise-induced asthma. (FALSE)

10. Diabetics should carry a carbohydrate snack with them when they exercise. (TRUE)

11. Aerobic exercise burns carbohydrates and fat. (TRUE)

12. The lactic acid system is a form of aerobic metabolism. (FALSE)

13. Doing curl-ups will take fat off the abdominals. (FALSE)

14. People who were athletes have less risk of disease even after they stop exercising. (FALSE)

Short Answer/Essay

1. Discuss the benefits of physical wellness or one of the five dimensions of wellness.

2. Name and define the five health-related components of physical fitness.

3. Describe the trends in physical activity/exercise over the past forty years.

4. What are the skill-related components of fitness and how do they impact health?

5. How much physical activity is enough?

6. Describe either aerobic or anaerobic metabolism.

7. Give an example of a specific, measurable goal.

8. What are the components of a physical activity session?

9. Select one physical activity principle and give an example of it at work.

Cardiorespiratory Endurance

Multiple Choice

1. Which of the following is FALSE?
   a. Most people prefer aerobic training over anaerobic training.
   b. Anaerobic training requires bouts of high intensity activity.
   c. Anaerobic training provides the cardiorespiratory base needed for recreational and daily activities.
   d. Anaerobic training is more performance oriented than aerobic training.

   answer: C(2)

2. The resting heart rate:
   a. generally decreases as fitness improves
   b. is influenced by stress, illness, and caffeine
   c. is counted after lying still for 30 minutes
   d. all of the above

   answer: D(2)

3. Cardiac output is a product of:
   a. stroke volume and heart rate
   b. stroke volume and ventilation rate
   c. heart rate and ventilation rate
   d. heart rate and oxygen consumption

   answer: A(1)

4. Stroke volume is the amount of blood:
   a. circulated through the body in one minute
   b. ejected from the heart per beat
   c. in the body
   d. the heart can hold in all four chambers

   answer: B(2)

5. Which of the following is an exercise training effect?
   a. the stroke volume of the heart increases
   b. the walls of the left ventricle become thicker
   c. the heart muscle becomes stronger
   d. all of the above

   answer: D(2)

6. Having a good network of capillaries can help prevent:
   a. stroke
   b. heart attack
   c. ischemia
   d. all of the above

   answer D(2)

7. Systolic blood pressure _____ during exercise.
   a. rises
   b. falls
   c. stays the same
   d. falls and then rises

   answer: A(2)

8. Regular exercise can result in:
   a. a decrease in blood plasma
   b. an increase in hemoglobin
   c. an increase in blood viscosity
   d. all of the above

   answer: B(2)

9. Which of the following is NOT a benefit of regular exercise?
   a. an increase in pulmonary ventilation
   b. an increase in mitochondria
   c. a decrease in stored glycogen
   d. all of the above

   answer: C(2)

10. Aerobic metabolism occurs in the:
    a. mitochondria
    b. cell cytoplasm
    c. motor neuron
    d. blood plasma

    answer: A(2)

11. The majority of health benefits received from regular aerobic exercise occur when a person exercises a minimum of _____ days a week.
    a. one to two
    b. two to four
    c. three to five
    d. six to seven

    answer: C(2)

12. Which of the following is NOT a benefit of regular aerobic exercise?
    a. decreased secretion of stress hormones
    b. alleviation of some depression
    c. insomnia
    d. release for pent up feelings

    answer: C(2)

13. Exercise addiction is characterized by all of the following EXCEPT:
    a. overuse injury
    b. putting exercise before family
    c. an increased resting heart rate
    d. malnutrition

    answer: D(2)

14. The threshold of training is the intensity at which:
    a. aerobic activity becomes anaerobic
    b. aerobic conditioning begin
    c. lactic acid build up becomes uncomfortable
    d. all of the above

    answer: B(2)

15. Heart rate's relationship to oxygen consumption is:
    a. almost linear
    b. curvilinear
    c. elliptical
    d. there is no relationship

    answer: A(1)

16. Aerobic conditioning occurs when exercise is performed within the:
    a. target heart rate minus age
    b. age-adjusted maximal heart rate
    c. target heart rate range
    d. maximum heart rate range

    answer: C(2)

17. Which of the following ranges is recommended for aerobic training?
    a. 60–80 percent of HRR
    b. 60–80 percent of VO2max
    c. 70–85 percent of MHR
    d. all of the above

    answer: D(2)

18. Using the Karvonen formula, what is the target heart rate zone for a 20-year-old with a resting heart rate of 50 beats per minute?
    a. 90–120 beats per minute
    b. 140–170 beats per minute
    c. 152–186 beats per minute
    d. 155–178 beats per minute

    answer: B(3)

19. Using a 70-85% range with the Maximum Heart Rate formula, the THR for a 20-year-old would be:
    a. 120–170 beats per minute
    b. 125–175 beats per minute
    c. 130–185 beats per minute
    d. 140–170 beats per minute

    answer: D(3)

20. The exercise heart rate (EHR) should be taken:
    a. before, during, and after class
    b. within 15 seconds after you stop exercising
    c. only at the carotid site
    d. several times during the aerobic session

    answer: D(2)

21. During exercise, the pulse should be counted for a period of:
    a. 6 seconds
    b. 10 seconds
    c. 15 seconds
    d. 30 seconds

    answer: B(1)

22. The carotid pulse is taken at the:
    a. wrist
    b. forehead
    c. neck
    d. thumb

    answer: C(1)

23. Intensity of exercise can be measured using:
    a. the talk test
    b. ratings of perceived exertion
    c. oxygen consumption
    d. all of the above

    answer: D(2)

24. According to ACSM, the optimal duration of a cardiorespiratory workout is _____ minutes.
    a. 10–15
    b. 12–25
    c. 20–60
    d. 60–90

    answer: C(2)

25. Who will show the most dramatic improvements in cardiorespiratory fitness?
    a. a beginner
    b. an athlete
    c. a recreational runner
    d. a dancer

    answer: A(2)

26. Which of the following assesses cardiorespiratory fitness?
    a. skinfold technique
    b. one mile run
    c. sit-and-reach
    d. underwater weighing

    answer: B(1)

27. Good hydration is important in:
    a. hot, humid weather
    b. cold weather
    c. high altitude activity
    d. all of the above

    answer: D(2)

True/False

1. Aerobic means "with oxygen." (TRUE)

2. Anaerobic activities are generally more than five minutes in duration. (FALSE)

3. A beginner should increase frequency and duration before increasing intensity. (TRUE)

4. The average resting heart rate is 50–60 beats per minute. (FALSE)

5. Healthy arteries are flexible. (TRUE)

6. Anaerobic processes take place in the cytoplasm of the muscle cell. (TRUE)

7. ATP and CP are high energy phosphagens. (TRUE)

8. Anaerobic training results in an increased storage of glycogen and high-energy phosphagens in the muscle. (TRUE)

9. The I in FIT stands for individuality. (FALSE)

10. Fifty percent of VO2max is the threshold of training. (TRUE)

11. If the exercise heart rate is above the target zone, a person is not exercising hard enough. (FALSE)

12. Ratings of perceived exertion are useful when heart rate is influenced by medication. (TRUE)

13. Aerobic activities more than an hour long bring diminishing returns in terms of health benefits. (TRUE)

14. Alcohol and sleeping pills may make altitude sickness worse. (TRUE)

15. Most people prefer anaerobic training to aerobic training. (FALSE)

Short Answer/Essay

1. Describe five health benefits associated with cardiorespiratory activity.

2. How is the heart influenced by cardiorespiratory training?

3. What is exercise's role in the prevention of arterial disease?

4. Distinguish between aerobic and anaerobic metabolism and explain how exercise affects both.

5. Calculate a training heart rate range for a 22 year old with a resting heart rate of 65 bpm.

6. Describe the procedure for taking the pulse.

7. Name four ways that exercise intensity can be monitored.

8. How hard, how long, and how often should a person exercise to develop cardiorespiratory fitness?

9. What precautions does a person need to take when exercising in the heat, cold, or high altitude?

Flexibility

Chapter 4

Multiple Choice

1. Flexibility refers to the range:
   a. in the strength of a muscle
   b. in the density of a bone
   c. of motion around a joint
   d. in volume of the lungs

   answer: C(2)

2. The range of motion through which a joint can move is limited by:
   a. musculotendinous structures
   b. ligamentous structures
   c. boney structures
   d. all of the above

   answer: D(2)

3. Connective tissue is NOT characterized by being:
   a. elastic and plastic
   b. hard and protective
   c. tough and fibrous
   d. binding and supportive

   answer: B(2)

4. Which of the following is NOT made up of connective tissue?
   a. bones
   b. muscle fascia
   c. tendons
   d. joint capsules

   answer: A(2)

5. Bones are bound to bones at articulations by:
   a. ligaments
   b. tendons
   c. muscles
   d. bursa sacks

   answer: A(1)

6. Synovial fluid lubricates:
   a. the heart
   b. joints
   c. the kidney
   d. none of the above

   answer: B(1)

7. To improve flexibility, the best thing to lengthen is:
   a. bone
   b. muscle
   c. tendon
   d. ligament

   answer: B(2)

8. Which of the following is NOT an influencing factor for flexibility?
   a. age
   b. physical activity
   c. hydration level
   d. muscle temperature

   answer: C(2)

9. Joint flexibility may be limited due to:
    a. injury or disease
    b. a person's height
    c. muscle boundness
    d. all of the above

    answer: A(2)

10. Low back pain can be the result of:
    a. weak abdominal muscles
    b. poor leg flexibility
    c. a sedentary lifestyle
    d. all of the above

    answer: D(2)

11. An "s" or "c" curvature of the spine is a characteristic of:
    a. scoliosis
    b. kyphosis
    c. lordosis
    d. none of the above

    answer: A(1)

12. Rounding of the upper back is characteristic of:
    a. scoliosis
    b. kyphosis
    c. lordosis
    d. none of the above

    answer: B(1)

13. A stretch reflex:
    a. is evoked by a static stretching
    b. is a voluntary motor response
    c. is controlled by muscle spindles
    d. results in decreased muscle tension

    answer: C(2)

14. Contracting one muscle in order to relax and stretch the opposing muscle is an example of:
    a. the stretch reflex
    b. an inverse myotatic reflex
    c. reciprocal innervation
    d. none of the above

    answer: C(2)

15. Static stretching:
    a. should be preceded by a general warm-up
    b. elicits a strong stretch reflex
    c. may stimulate the Golgi tendon organ
    d. uses a bounce-type action

    answer: C(2)

16. Static stretching should be held for a minimum of _____ seconds.
    a. 5
    b. 10
    c. 30
    d. 60

    answer: B(1)

17. During passive stretching:
    a. a series of isometric contractions and stretches is performed
    b. an outside force acts to put the muscle in stretch
    c. one muscle contracts while the other relaxes
    d. all of the above

    answer: B(2)

18. In an active stretch:
    a. a partner places you in a stretch position
    b. the opposing muscle is contracted
    c. an outside force acts to put the muscle in stretch
    d. isometric and concentric contractions of the opposing muscle are performed

    answer: B(2)

19. Which of the following is the most effective form of stretching?
    a. static
    b. ballistic
    c. PNF
    d. active static

    answer: C(2)

20. Which of the following has the disadvantage of taking longer and causing more muscle soreness?
    a. PNF stretching
    b. static stretching
    c. active stretching
    d. ballistic stretching

    answer: A(2)

21. Flexibility can be maintained by stretching a minimum of _____ days a week.
    a. one
    b. two
    c. three
    d. four

    answer: C(2)

22. A good field test for low back and hamstring flexibility is the:
    a. curl-up test
    b. push-up test
    c. step test
    d. sit-and-reach test

    answer: D(1)

True/False

1. Joints can have ranges of motion in more than one direction. (TRUE)

2. Flexibility can be developed at any age. (TRUE)

3. Girls are more flexible than boys. (TRUE)

4. The rapid lengthening of the muscle during ballistic stretching elicits the stretch reflex. (TRUE)

5. Men have traditionally selected physical activities that require flexibility more often than women. (FALSE)

6. Low-back pain is usually the result of weak abdominal muscles and poor leg and hip flexibility. (TRUE)

7. A cramp can be relieved by placing the opposing muscle in contraction. (FALSE)

8. The cervical curve is the lower curvature of the spine. (FALSE)

9. Functional scoliosis is the result of an inherited trait. (FALSE)

10. Kyphosis is better known as sway back. (FALSE)

11. Static stretching quiets the stretch reflex and takes advantage of the relaxation signals of the Golgi tendon organ. (TRUE)

12. A good stretching regimen is to hold a stretch for 20 - 60 seconds, several times. (TRUE)

13. A stretch should be done to the point of discomfort but not pain. (TRUE)

14. PNF stretching was developed for rehabilitative purposes. (TRUE)

Short Answer/Essay

1. Define flexibility.

2. Discuss the benefits of good flexibility.

3. Identify the strengths and weaknesses of static, ballistic, and PNF stretching.

4. Identify three factors that influence flexibility and explain their influence.

5. What is the procedure for relieving a cramp?

6. Explain how flexibility is related to low-back pain.

7. Explain the stretching implications of the stretch reflex, inverse myotatic reflex, and reciprocal innervation.

8. Explain the difference between passive and active stretching.

9. Apply the FIT principle to flexibility.

Muscular Strength and Endurance

TEST BANK Chapter 5

Multiple Choice

1. Muscular strength is
   a. the number of times a muscle can repeatedly contract against a force
   b. the maximum amount of force a muscle can exert against a resistance one time
   c. the length of time a muscle can hold a contraction without fatigue
   d. none of the above

   answer B(2)

2. Muscular endurance is NOT:
   a. closely related but distinct from muscular strength
   b. the ability to exert a submaximal force repeatedly
   c. the ability to maintain a submaximal force for a period of time
   d. the maximum force a muscle can exert

   answer D(2)

3. Which of the following involves a competition of several lifts with as much weight as possible:
   a. body sculpting
   b. weight training
   c. weight lifting
   d. resistance training

   answer C(2)

4. Which of the following is composed of myofibers?
   a. fiber
   b. myofiber
   c. myofilament
   d. sarcomere

   answer A(1)

5. Resistance training results in all of the following EXCEPT:
   a. less tolerance to lactic acid
   b. more ATP and PC stored in the muscle
   c. the ability to do more work with less fatigue
   d. all of the above

   answer C(2)

6. A motor unit consists of a:
   a. motor neuron and a motor endplate
   b. sensory neuron and a motor endplate
   c. motor neuron and muscle fibers
   d. motor endplate and muscle fibers

   answer C(1)

7. To recruit more muscle fibers, perform:
   a. a high number of consecutive repetitions
   b. more than one set of repetitions
   c. two exercises in a row that work the same muscle
   d. all of the above

   answer D(2)

8. Which of the following is TRUE of slow twitch fibers?
   a. they respond most to aerobic training
   b. they respond most to anaerobic training
   c. they have a greater capacity to store ATP and CP than fast twitch fibers
   d. b and c

   answer A(2)

9. Slow twitch muscle fibers _____ than fast twitch muscle fibers.
   a. have fewer mitochondria
   b. have more oxidative enzymes
   c. are more involved in anaerobic metabolism
   d. are better at extracting oxygen from the blood

   answer C(2)

10. The structural unit of a muscle fiber is:
    a. an actin myofilament
    b. a myosin myofilament
    c. a sarcomere
    d. a chain of ATP

    answer C(1)

11. When sarcomeres shorten, all of the following happen EXCEPT:
    a. the muscle visibly lengthens
    b. the actin myofilaments slide over the myosin myofilaments
    c. a concentric contraction occurs
    d. the angle of an involved joint is changed

    answer A(2)

12. During an eccentric contraction, the muscle:
    a. lengthens against a resistance
    b. shortens against a resistance
    c. shortens over a range of motion
    d. maintains tension in one position

    answer A(2)

13. To develop strength throughout a range of motion, use all of the following types of contraction except:
    a. concentric
    b. isometric
    c. isotonic
    d. isokinetic

    answer B(1)

14. During a(n) _____ contraction, tension is varied while speed is held constant.
    a. isometric
    b. concentric
    c. isokinetic
    d. eccentric

    answer C(2)

15. Strength (power) training is characterized by a _____ amount of resistance and a _____ number of repetitions.
    a. high, low
    b. low, high
    c. high, high
    d. low, low

    answer A(2)

16. Strength training of a muscle or group of muscles should be performed:
    a. every day
    b. once a week
    c. on alternate days
    d. five times a week

    answer C(2)

17. Which of the following is NOT true about muscle hypertrophy?
    a. Muscle hypertrophy occurs more often in men than women.
    b. Muscle hypertrophy mainly involves slow twitch fibers.
    c. Strength gains can occur without simultaneous muscle hypertrophy.
    d. Muscle hypertrophy is the increasing of muscle cell size.

    answer B(2)

18. The Valsalva Maneuver is characterized by all of the following EXCEPT:
    a. holding the breath and contracting the chest muscles
    b. an increase in thoracic pressure
    c. difficulty swallowing while exercising
    d. dizziness and/or light headedness

    answer C(2) .

19. Muscles used for gross motor movement have _____ muscle fibers associated with each motor unit, than muscles used for fine motor movement.
    a. more
    b. fewer
    c. the same number of
    d. an indeterminate number of

    answer A(2)

20. Which arm position creates the greatest overload during a curl-up?
    a. arms bent and held near the head
    b. arms extended overhead
    c. arms folded across the chest
    d. arms alongside the body

    answer B(2)

21. Weight training may by contraindicated (harmful) for people:
    a. with high blood pressure
    b. with arthritic joints
    c. with tendinitis
    d. all of the above

    answer D(2)

22. Which of the following is a test of muscular endurance?
    a. one mile walk/run test
    b. sit-up (curl-up) test
    c. skinfold test
    d. sit-and-reach test

    answer B(1)

23. Which of the following is FALSE?
    a. A large increase in intensity can result in delayed-muscle soreness.
    b. Women's muscles will respond to strength work by increasing in size.
    c. Muscles push and pull to achieve concentric and eccentric contractions.
    d. all of the above

    answer C(2)

24. Squats do NOT work the _____ muscle(s).
    a. trapezius
    b. quadriceps
    c. hamstring
    d. gluteal

    answer A(1)

25. Curl-ups work which of the following muscle(s)?
    a. quadriceps
    b. gluteals
    c. rectus abdominus
    d. spinae erectors

    answer C(1)

26. Which of the following exercises should be avoided in a health-related workout?
    a. deep knee bends
    b. head rolls to the front and side
    c. single leg lifts
    d. all of the above

    answer A(2)

27. Hypertrophy refers to an increase in:
    a. weight
    b. muscle size
    c. stamina
    d. bone density

    answer B(2)

28. Isotonic means equal:
    a. length
    b. tension
    c. speed
    d. diameter

    answer B(1)

29. Which of the following muscles is responsible for the rotation in a twisting curl-up?
    a. rectus abdominus
    b. transversalis
    c. spinal erectors
    d. obliques

    answer D(1)

30. During a curl-up, the:
    a. low back should press into the floor
    b. neck should be pulled forward
    c. knees should be kept straight
    d. none of the above

    answer A(2)

31. Which of the following statements is FALSE?
    a. men's muscles generate more force per square centimeter of cross section
    b. men and women hypertrophy at the same rate
    c. women's muscles will, with training, become as large as a man's
    d. men and women have similar relative strengths

    answer C(2)

32. Anabolic steroids:
    a. increase muscle size
    b. a dangerous to your health
    c. are illegal to buy
    d. all of the above

    answer D(2)

33. Free weights are:
    a. machine weights
    b. dumbbells and barbells
    c. promotional weights
    d. none of the above

    answer C(1)

34. Free weights provide a:
    a. constant resistance
    b. variable resistance
    c. multidirectional resistance
    d. balanced resistance

    answer A(2)

35. An arm-curl is an example of:
    a. isometric contraction
    b. dynamic contraction
    c. eccentric contraction
    d. static contraction

    answer B(2)

36. Pushing as hard as you can against something that doesn't move is a(n):
    a. isotonic contraction
    b. isometric contraction
    c. isokinetic contraction
    d. isomorphic contraction

    answer B(2)

37. For general fitness, perform resistance exercises _____ a week.
    a. once
    b. two or three times
    c. four times
    d. five times

    answer B(2)

38. To develop endurance, take breaks of _____ seconds between sets.
    a. 10–30 seconds
    b. 30–60 seconds
    c. 60–90 seconds
    d. 90–20 seconds

    answer A(2)

39. Power is a combination of:
    a. strength and endurance
    b. strength and speed
    c. endurance and speed
    d. strength, endurance, and speed

    answer B(1)

40. A strength workout is fueled by:
    a. the phosphagen system
    b. lactic acid system
    c. aerobic system
    d. a and b

    answer D(2)

True/False

1. Wellness requires enough strength and endurance to handle daily activities, leisure activities, and emergencies. (TRUE)

2. Pushing a car out of a ditch is an example of muscular strength and power. (TRUE)

3. Very few repetitions with heavy weights will produce muscle hypertrophy. (FALSE)

4. Muscular strength and endurance programs are not recommended for most older adults. (FALSE)

5. Pulling against the water in a pool is a form of resistance training. (TRUE)

6. Muscular endurance can be developed dynamically or statically. (TRUE)

41. One set of 10 RM means to perform 10 repetitions:
    a. using a maximum load
    b. with enough resistance to cause fatigue by lift number 10
    c. with light weights
    d. b and c

    answer B(2)

42. Which of the following is NOT true about circuit resistance training:
    a. it is not a substitute for aerobic training
    b. it can be performed using free weights or machines
    c. it can be done in mini-circuits
    d. it takes longer to perform than most other resistance type programs

    answer D(2)

7. Body building is a contest of muscle size, symmetry, and definition. (TRUE)

8. Weight training is detrimental to athletes who need speed. (FALSE)

9. Resistance training is primarily aerobic. (FALSE)

10. A marathon run depends primarily upon slow twitch fibers. (TRUE)

11. The amount of slow and fast twitch fibers a person has is genetically determined. (TRUE)

12. Strength training will produce endurance gains. (TRUE)

13. Women have the same absolute strength as men but less relative strength. (FALSE)

14. Anabolic steroids do not help increase muscle mass. (FALSE)

15. The length of a workout is determined by the number of repetitions, sets, and length of breaks. (TRUE)

Short Answer/Essay

1. Select five of the following terms to define: muscular strength, muscular endurance, weight training, resistance training, weight lifting, body building and body sculpting.

2. How much strength and endurance does a person need?

3. What are the benefits of having good muscular strength and endurance?

4. Describe the anatomy and physiology of a muscle.

5. Discuss gender differences in strength and endurance training and effect.

6. Describe two of the following types of programs using the FIT Principle: general fitness, power, hypertrophy, strength, endurance.

7. Define and give an example of an isokinetic, isometric, and isotonic contraction.

8. Identify 10 exercises a person could do to get a good general strength/endurance workout.

Multiple Choice

1. Which of the following factors influences a person's choice of foods?
    a. time of day
    b. what food looks like
    c. what parents eat
    d. all of the above

    answer: D(1)

2. Poor food choices or overeating may cause all of the following, EXCEPT:
    a. heart disease
    b. liver disease
    c. cancer
    d. arthritis

    answer: D(2)

3. The base of the food pyramid is made of:
    a. vegetable group
    b. milk, yogurt, cheese group
    c. bread, cereal, rice, and pasta group
    d. meat, poultry, fish, dried beans, eggs, and nuts group

    answer: C(1)

4. The recommended number of servings of fruits for adults per day is:
    a. 2–4
    b. 3–5
    c. 5–8
    d. 8–11

    answer: A(1)

5. The recommended number of servings of vegetables for adults per day is:
    a. 2–4
    b. 3–5
    c. 4–8
    d. 6–11

    answer: B(1)

6. The recommended number of servings of bread and cereals for adults per day is:
    a. 2–4
    b. 3–6
    c. 8–10
    d. 6–11

    answer: D(1)

7. RDA stands for:
    a. recommended dietary allowances
    b. red dye additive
    c. regulatory daily allowance
    d. resource dietary assistance

    answer: A(1)

8. The recommended diet for a normal healthy adult is one which includes:
    a. less than 30% fat
    b. 30% to 40% carbohydrate
    c. 10–12% carbohydrate
    d. 58–60% protein

    answer: A(1)

220

9. Carbohydrate, fat, and protein produce _____, _____, and _____ kilocalories of energy per gram respectively.
   a. 10, 6, 5
   b. 5, 10, 6
   c. 9, 4, 4
   d. 4, 9, 4

   answer: D(1)

10. Fat is a necessary component of proper nutrition because it:
    a. helps to insulate and protect vital organs and tissues
    b. provides storage for several fat-soluble vitamins
    c. is an efficient storehouse of energy
    d. all of the above

    answer: D(2)

11. Which of the following takes the least energy to store:
    a. carbohydrates
    b. fat
    c. protein
    d. vitamins

    answer: B(2)

12. The six basic nutrients are:
    a. protein, water, fiber, vitamins, carbohydrate, fat
    b. protein, water, fat, vitamins, carbohydrate, minerals
    c. carbohydrate, fat, water, fiber, vitamins, minerals
    d. vitamins, minerals, fat, protein, fiber, carbohydrate

    answer: B(1)

13. Which of the following types of triglycerides has all the hydrogen atoms it can hold?
    a. monounsaturated
    b. polyunsaturated
    c. saturated
    d. phospholipids

    answer: C(2)

14. Members of the fat family include:
    a. glucose, sucrose, and starch
    b. triglycerides and cholesterol
    c. amino acids and peptides
    d. all of the above

    answer: B(1)

15. Polyunsaturated fats:
    a. are made up of lipids and cholesterol
    b. are solids at room temperature
    c. help keep blood cholesterol levels low
    d. come from animal sources

    answer: C(2)

16. Saturated fat is NOT:
    a. directly related to heart disease
    b. used by the liver to produce cholesterol
    c. found in corn and peanut oil
    d. good tasting in foods and used as a thickener

    answer: C(2)

17. Members of the carbohydrate family include:
    a. glucose, sucrose, and starch
    b. triglycerides and cholesterol
    c. amino acids and peptides
    d. riboflavin and niacin

    answer: A(1)

18. Which of the following is the primary source of energy for all human metabolism?
    a. fat
    b. protein
    c. vitamins
    d. carbohydrates

    answer: D(1)

19. Natural occurring sugars are found in:
    a. fruits
    b. vegetables
    c. milk
    d. all of the above

    answer: D(2)

20. Empty calorie foods include:
    a. refined sugars
    b. fruits and vegetables
    c. milk
    d. none of the above

    answer: A(1)

21. Carbohydrates:
    a. are broken down into simple sugars
    b. are stored as glycogen in the liver and muscle tissue
    c. are the main fuel for intense physical activity
    d. all of the above

    answer: D(2)

22. Complex carbohydrates:
    a. come from plant sources
    b. are low in calories and high in nutrients
    c. are made up of long complex chains of simple sugars
    d. all of the above

    answer: D(2)

23. Which of the following foods is a good source of antioxidants?
    a. broccoli
    b. milk
    c. fish
    d. nuts

    answer: A(1)

24. Which of the following is NOT a source of energy?
    a. fiber
    b. protein
    c. fat
    d. carbohydrate

    answer: A(1)

25. Which of the following adds bulk to food in the intestine?
    a. fat
    b. protein
    c. fiber
    d. carbohydrate

    answer: C(1)

26. Which of the following foods is NOT a good source of fiber?
    a. bran
    b. popcorn
    c. dried beans
    d. cheese

    answer: D(1)

27. Fiber reduces the risk of all of the following EXCEPT:
    a. diverticulitis
    b. high blood cholesterol
    c. heart disease
    d. cancer

    answer: B(2)

28. A complete protein is one that:
    a. contains all the essential amino acids
    b. is derived entirely from plant sources
    c. is made up of complex carbohydrates
    d. contains all the necessary vitamins

    answer: A(2)

29. Protein does all of the following EXCEPT:
    a. aids in the growth and structure of body tissues
    b. supplies energy to muscles for movement
    c. forms important parts of hormones
    d. provides shock absorption for the internal organs

    answer: D(2)

30. Which of the following contains all nine essential amino acids?
    a. poultry
    b. vegetables
    c. fish
    d. red meats

    answer: D(2)

31. Athletes who wish to build muscle mass need the greatest increase in:
    a. protein
    b. carbohydrate
    c. fat
    d. fiber

    answer: B(3)

32. Which of the following types of vegetarians will not eat meat and eggs but will eat dairy products?
    a. vegans
    b. lactovegetarians
    c. lacto-ovo-vegetarians
    d. b and c

    answer: B(1)

33. Vitamins:
    a. help release energy from the foods we eat
    b. by themselves produce energy
    c. provide all the nutrients you need to be healthy
    d. need protein in order to dissolve

    answer: A(2)

34. Vitamins:
    a. can be manufactured by the body in small amounts
    b. function as metabolic regulators
    c. are inorganic in nature
    d. are a limited source of calories

    answer: B(2)

35. Which of the following is NOT true about vitamins A, D, E, and K?
    a. are fat-soluble
    b. need to be consumed daily
    c. can be toxic in big doses
    d. can be stored

    answer: B(2)

36. Consuming a vitamin in a dose in excess of 10 times its RDA is called:
    a. shooting up
    b. overdosing
    c. megadosing
    d. carbo loading

    answer: C(1)

37. Which of the following people is LEAST likely to need vitamin supplements?
    a. a pregnant or lactating woman
    b. a person on a medically supervised low-calorie diet
    c. a physically active person eating a well balanced diet
    d. an elderly person who does not consume a balanced diet

    answer: C(2)

38. Free radicals:
    a. are oxygen molecules that have lost one too many electrons
    b. may be responsible for premature aging, cancer, and heart disease
    c. are reduced when they meet another free radical or an antioxidant
    d. all of the above

    answer: D(2)

39. Which of the following vitamins are believed to act as antioxidants?
    a. A, D, E, K
    b. A, C, E
    c. B, B-12, C
    d. B, D, C

    answer: B(1)

40. Which of the following are all major minerals?
    a. chloride, calcium, iron, zinc
    b. calcium, phosphorus, magnesium, sodium
    c. magnesium, copper, sodium, iodine
    d. calcium, magnesium, zinc, selenium

    answer: B(1)

41. A deficiency in calcium may result in:
    a. osteoporosis
    b. diabetes
    c. anemia
    d. cancer

    answer: A(1)

42. Which of the following is the best food source of calcium?
    a. citrus juice
    b. organ meats
    c. whole wheat grains
    d. leafy green vegetables

    answer: D(1)

43. A deficiency in iron can result in:
    a. amenorrhea
    b. anemia
    c. osteoporosis
    d. asthma

    answer: B(2)

44. Which of the following would probably contain the LEAST sodium?
    a. processed foods
    b. dried or smoked meats
    c. fast foods
    d. fresh vegetables

    answer: D(1)

45. The estimated minimum daily requirement of sodium for healthy adults is:
    a. 100–1,000 mg
    b. 500–1,200 mg
    c. 1,100–3,000 mg
    d. 3,200–5,000 mg

    answer: C(1)

46. Water is a nutrient for which all of the following are true EXCEPT:
    a. helps maintain cellular fluid balance
    b. helps regulate body temperature
    c. acts as a solvent for other nutrients
    d. should be taken in small quantities during weight loss

    answer: D(2)

47. The body needs approximately ____ cups of fluid a day.
    a. 4
    b. 8
    c. 10
    d. 12

    answer: B(1)

48. Which of the following statements about fast food is FALSE?
    a. one out of five Americans eats at a fast-food restaurant each day
    b. fast foods tend to be high in fiber and complex carbohydrates
    c. careful selection of fast foods can result in a nutritious meal
    d. restaurants will sell what the public wants to eat

    answer: B(2)

49. If a food label says a food has 7 grams of fat and a total of 100 calories, what percentage of the calories are fat calories?
    a. 7 %
    b. 28 %
    c. 63 %
    d. 70%

    answer: C(3)

50. Which of the following statements is FALSE?
    a. people who are physically active require a higher fluid intake
    b. sport drinks offer no advantage over water for a normally active person
    c. sport drinks may benefit people involved in prolonged endurance activities
    d. most sport drinks are absorbed into the body more quickly than plain cool water

    answer: B(2)

51. Carbohydrate loading does NOT:
    a. increase the storage of glycogen in the muscles and liver
    b. allow a person to be physically active longer with less fatigue
    c. benefit persons involved in moderate intensity activities lasting 20–60 minutes
    d. involve a gradual reduction of physical activity and increase in carbohydrate consumption four days before an event

    answer: C(3)

52. The best diet is one which is
    a. high in protein
    b. low in carbohydrate
    c. low in fat
    d. all of the above

    answer: C(1)

True/False

1. There is a close relationship between the amount of fat a person eats and the amount of body fat a person possesses. (TRUE)

2. Fats are made up of glycerol and fatty acids. (TRUE)

3. Saturated fats are solids at room temperature. (TRUE)

4. Palm and coconut oil contain saturated fat. (TRUE)

5. Polyunsaturated fat is linked with high blood cholesterol. (FALSE)

6. Diets high in fat are linked to heart disease, diabetes, and cancer. (TRUE)

7. One gram of fat contains a total of four grams of available energy. (FALSE)

8. Complementary incomplete proteins eaten together at the same meal provide all the essential amino acids. (TRUE)

9. Most of the diseases linked with diet in the United States are the result of malnutrition. (FALSE)

10. The most readily absorbed iron comes from plant foods as opposed to animal foods. (FALSE)

11. Processed foods tend to be high in sodium and fat. (TRUE)

12. Approximately 35 percent of the adult population in the industrialized world are considered obese. (TRUE)

13. About 50 percent of the adults in the United States are considered overweight. (TRUE)

14. Muscular people burn more calories at rest than less muscular people. (TRUE)

15. A high protein diet can result in dehydration. (TRUE)

16. A starvation diet may result in an increase in metabolic rate. (TRUE)

17. Men tend to suffer an iron deficiency more often than women. (FALSE)

18. Research has found that about half of adults are salt sensitive enough to cause high blood pressure. (FALSE)

19. Thirst is a good indicator of dehydration. (FALSE)

Short Answer/Essay

1. Describe five factors that influence food choices.

2. How is the food pyramid different from what has been recommended in the past?

3. Describe three functions of fat. carbohydrates, and protein. (total of nine functions)

4. What are the dangers of being obese?

5. Describe five ways you can cut down on dietary fat.

6. Describe five ways you can cut down on sodium.

Multiple Choice

1. Body length and shape are largely determined by:
    a. heredity
    b. diet
    c. physical activity
    d. all of the above

    answer: A (1)

2. Fat weight is largely determined by:
    a. heredity
    b. diet
    c. physical activity
    d. all of the above

    answer: D(2)

3. Body fat:
    a. pads organs
    b. provides fuel for movement
    c. insulates the body
    d. all of the above

    answer: D(1)

4. What amount of body fat is essential for men and women respectively?
    a. 5 % men, 12% women
    b. 10% men, 18% women
    c. 12% men, 15% women
    d. 15% men, 20% women

    answer: A(1)

5. Which of the following is not a type of body fat?
    a. cellulite
    b. coagulated
    c. intramuscular
    d. subcutaneous

    answer: B(1)

6. Too little essential fat may result in all of the following EXCEPT:
    a. hypoglycemia
    b. lower calcium absorption
    c. bone density loss
    d. amenorrhea

    answer: A(2)

7. Which of the following is more TRUE of men than women?
    a. they need more essential fat
    b. they tend to store fat in the abdomen, chest and back
    c. cellulite is more apparent
    d. all of the above

    answer: B(2)

8. Each gram of fat has _____ calories available for muscle contraction or other metabolic processes.
    a. four
    b. five
    c. seven
    d. nine

    answer: D(1)

9. Percent body fat is all of the following EXCEPT:
   a. the amount of total weight that is fat
   b. a good indicator of health risk
   c. the amount of subcutaneous fat a person has
   d. a better indicator of health risk than weight

   answer: C(2)

10. Men and women are considered obese starting at _____ percent fat.
    a. 15 % for men, 18 % for women
    b. 20 % for men, 25 % for women
    c. 25 % for men, 32 % for women
    d. 32 % for men, 38 % for women

    answer: C(1)

11. It is possible to be:
    a. overweight and at a healthy or lean percentage of fat
    b. an "ideal weight" and be overfat
    c. a different weight than someone else but have the same percentage of fat
    d. all of the above

    answer: D(3)

12. An android body type is characterized by all of the following EXCEPT:
    a. an apple shape
    b. excess upper body fat
    c. more common among women than men
    d. associated with greater risk of heart disease, cancer, and diabetes

    answer: C(2)

13. Abdominal fat
    a. is associated with a higher incidence of disease than leg fat
    b. cells are larger than other fat cells and have an intolerance for blood sugars and insulin
    c. is easily stored and released which can lead to a rise in blood cholesterol
    d. all of the above

    answer: D(3)

14. Excessive leanness may be due to:
    a. an eating disorder
    b. a very low-calorie restricted diet
    c. regular prolonged endurance-type activities
    d. all of the above

    answer: D(2)

15. Which of the following is the "healthy" range for percentage fat?
    a. 8–15 % for men; 13–20 % for women
    b. 10–20 % for men; 18–25 % for women
    c. 14–26 % for men; 20–28 % for women
    d. 18–25 % for men; 25–32 % for women

    answer: B(1)

16. Obese individuals have an elevated risk of all of the following EXCEPT:
    a. high blood pressure
    b. high blood cholesterol
    c. testosterone
    d. premature death

    answer: C(1)

17. Obesity may result in:
    a. guilt
    b. discrimination
    c. low self-esteem
    d. all of the above

    answer: D(1)

18. Which of the following is NOT a method of assessing body fat?
    a. hydrostatic (underwater) weighing
    b. skinfold technique
    c. bioelectric impedance
    d. stepping on a scale

    answer: D(2)

19. Hydrostatic weighing involves which of the following?
    a. lowering a person sitting on a scale into a tank of water
    b. taking fat measurements on the back, arm, and hip
    c. lowering a person into a tank of water with weights added to make sure they sink
    d. sending electrical impulses through a fully hydrated person

    answer: A(1)

20. A percentage of body fat is calculated after using a bioelectric impedance machine to:
    a. measure the amount of resistance a small electrical charge meets as it travels through the body
    b. measure total body water based on the speed with which a small electrical charge travels through the body
    c. measure fat deposits by placing electrodes on various locations of the body and sending a small electrical signal into the deposits to measure their depth
    d. measure muscle mass based on the echowaves generated as a small electric charge travels through the body

    answer: A(2)

21. Common sites for skinfold measures are the:
    a. inside of the ankle, back of arm, top of shoulder, abdomen
    b. abdomen, back of arm, front of thigh, low back
    c. abdomen, back of arm, hip, below shoulder blade, thigh
    d. abdomen, front of the arm, back, calf

    answer: C(1)

True/False

1. Upper body fat is associated with more health risk than lower body fat. (TRUE)

2. Body length and shape are primarily determined through exercise. (FALSE)

3. Muscles, skin, and blood are classified as lean body mass. (TRUE)

4. Excessive nonessential fat is unhealthy. (TRUE)

5. Intramuscular fat is stored around the internal organs. (FALSE)

6. Cellulite is fat trapped in the connective tissue that attaches your skin to the underlying muscles. (TRUE)

7. Each gram of fat produces nine calories of energy. (TRUE)

8. Two people can be different weights and the same percentage of body fat. (TRUE)

9. A gynoid body type is described as pear shaped. (TRUE)

10. An android body shape is associated with a greater risk of heart disease, stroke, cancer, and diabetes than a gynoid body shape. (TRUE)

11. Most people are a combination of android and gynoid body shapes. (TRUE)

12. Android fat is easy to take on and off as compared to gynoid fat. (FALSE)

13. Hydrostatic weighing is the least effective measurement of body fat. (FALSE)

14. Bioelectric impedance measures subcutaneous fat. (FALSE)

15. Determining body fat requires knowledge of sophisticated, highly computerized equipment. (FALSE)

16. Determining percentage of body fat can help determine a person's ideal body weight. (TRUE)

17. Essential fat for a man is about five percent. (TRUE)

18. Essential fat for a woman is about 15 percent. (FALSE)

19. Some cellulite cannot be removed even with a proper diet and exercise. (TRUE)

20. Women with too little fat may develop amenorrhea (menstruation cessation). (TRUE)

21. High blood pressure is three times higher amongst the obese. (TRUE)

22. Obesity can lead to psychological stress. (TRUE)

Short Answer/Essay

1. Discuss the health risks of being overfat.

2. What determines the amount of fat weight a person has?

3. Where in the body is fat stored?

4. Discuss gender differences concerning the amount and placement of stored fat.

5. What are the main functions of fat?

6. How is body fat distributed, and how does this relate to disease?

7. What are some of the psychological impacts of obesity?

8. Compare and contrast methods of determining percent body fat.

9. Describe two methods of determining body shape and health risk.

10. If a person wants to lower his/her body fat, what would you tell him/her?

Controlling Body Weight

TEST BANK

Chapter **8**

Multiple Choice

1. Which of the following is FALSE?
   a. over one-half of men and three-quarters of women are unhappy with their current weight
   b. weight-loss is a multi-billion dollar industry
   c. fewer than one-half of the women who diet need to lose weight
   d. most women diet for health reasons

   answer: D(2)

2. What percentage of adult women are believed to be on a diet?
   a. 10–20 %
   b. 30–40 %
   c. 60–70 %
   d. 80–90 %

   answer: B(1)

3. If less energy is expended than taken in (as food), there is a
   a. calorie balance
   b. negative calorie balance
   c. tendency to gain weight
   d. tendency to maintain weight

   answer: C(2)

4. According to the set point theory:
   a. increased consumption results in a more efficient use of calories
   b. repeated bouts of dieting make it easier to lose weight
   c. the body strives to maintain a certain pre-determined percentage of fat
   d. during starvation the body uses calories more efficiently

   answer: C(2)

5. Resting metabolic rate (RMR) is influenced by:
   a. genetics
   b. rapid weight gains and losses
   c. exercise
   d. all of the above

   answer: D(1)

6. Which of the following statements concerning metabolic rate is FALSE?
   a. women tend to have a higher metabolic rate than men
   b. muscle mass increases resting metabolic rate
   c. metabolic rate increases with age
   d. stimulants like caffeine temporarily raise metabolic rate

   answer: C(2)

7. All of the following play a role in obesity EXCEPT:
   a. genetic factors
   b. cultural factors
   c. lifestyle factors
   d. intellectual factors

   answer: D(1)

8. Anorexia nervosa is characterized by all of the following EXCEPT:
   a. self-starvation through diet and exercise
   b. attention seeking behavior
   c. denial of weight loss
   d. malnutrition

   answer: B(1)

9. Bulimia is characterized by:
   a. binge and purge behavior
   b. self-starvation
   c. cessation of menstruation
   d. refusal to maintain normal body weight

   answer: A(1)

10. Which of the following diseases risks damage to the throat and esophagus?
    a. anorexia nervosa
    b. bulimia
    c. obesity
    d. all of the above

    answer: B(2)

11. Fat loss is maximized when a negative calorie balance is achieved through:
    a. diet alone
    b. exercise alone
    c. a combination of diet and exercise
    d. a combination of exercise and stress management

    answer: C(1)

12. Which of the following types of exercise is recommended for a weight-loss program?
    a. aerobic
    b. anaerobic
    c. aerodynamic
    d. acrobatic

    answer: A(2)

13. Exercise frequency for weight-loss purposes should be _____ days a week.
    a. 2–3
    b. 3–5
    c. 4–6
    d. 6–7

    answer: D(1)

14. After _____ minutes aerobic exercise burns approximately 50 percent fat.
    a. 12
    b. 20
    c. 30
    d. 45

    answer: B(1)

15. If a person loses 5 pounds of fat and puts on 5 pounds of muscle s/he will
    a. gain weight and lower percentage of fat
    b. lose weight and lower percentage of fat
    c. stay the same weight and lower percentage of fat
    d. stay the same weight and the same percentage of fat

    answer: C(3)

16. When dieting, total daily caloric intake should not be reduced more than _____ calories per day for a present diet under 3000 calories and should not be reduced more than _____ calories per day for a present diet over 3000 calories.
    a. 100, 1000
    b. 250, 500
    c. 500, 1000
    d. 1000, 1200

    answer: C(2)

17. Unless under medical supervision, a person should consume a minimum of _____ calories per day.
    a. 1,000
    b. 1,200
    c. 1,500
    d. 2,000

    answer: B(1)

18. Which is NOT a good habit for weight control?
    a. eliminating eating cues
    b. eating home-cooked meals rather than restaurant meals
    c. preplanning shopping lists
    d. eating two big meals a day and skipping breakfast

    answer: D(2)

19. Which of the following weight-loss plans is used with some obese individuals when normal diet methods fail?
    a. very low calorie diet (VLCD)
    b. yo-yo diet
    c. weight cycling diet
    d. none of the above

    answer: A(2)

True/False Questions

1. It is possible to be overweight and not be overfat. (TRUE)

20. Quick weight-loss in the first week usually represents a:
    a. loss of readily available fat stores
    b. loss of carbohydrate stores and the water stored with it
    c. temporary loss of muscle mass
    d. loss of fiber from the intestinal tract

    answer: B(3)

21. The recommended safe weight-loss is _____ pounds per week.
    a. 0.5–1
    b. 1–2
    c. 2–3
    d. 3–4

    answer: A(1)

22. Weight gain can be achieved through:
    a. a balanced diet and resistance exercise
    b. a balanced diet and aerobic exercise
    c. a high protein diet, low carbohydrate diet and resistance exercise
    d. a low fat diet and aerobic exercise

    answer: A(2)

23. In order to maintain a healthy weight, one must commit to:
    a. regular physical activity
    b. a balanced diet
    c. a plan of action in the event of a relapse
    d. all of the above

    answer: D(2)

2. Even moderate exercise makes dieting difficult because it increases your appetite. (FALSE)

3. The desire to be "thin" is fueled more by vanity and social acceptance than health. (TRUE)

4. Americans are the most overfat people in the world with one quarter of the population considered to be clinically obese. (TRUE)

5. The only effective way to lower the set point is through regular physical activity. (TRUE)

6. Metabolism is the sum of all the vital body processes by which food, energy, and nutrients are made available to, and used by the body. (TRUE)

7. Metabolic rate is influenced by genetics, age, illness, stimulants, and exercise. (TRUE)

8. Women generally have higher metabolic rates than men. (FALSE)

9. Children of obese parents are more apt to be obese than children of healthy weight parents. (TRUE)

10. People who wish to overcome an eating disorder need both medical and psychological treatment. (TRUE)

11. Men suffer from bulimia more often than women. (FALSE)

12. Exercise results in the body expending about 15 more calories for every 100 calories used during exercise. (TRUE)

13. The environmental, cultural and lifestyle factors that influence what and how we eat, as well as whether we are physically active, are the greatest causes of obesity. (TRUE)

14. Carbohydrate is more easily stored than fat or protein. (FALSE)

15. Safe and successful weight-loss strategies are achieved through a combination of a balanced diet and exercise. (TRUE)

16. A desirable weight-loss program according to the American College of Sports Medicine is one that has a diet consisting of no less than 800 calories. (FALSE)

17. The increase in body fat that occurs between age 20 and 60 is called age-onset obesity. (TRUE)

18. Each gram of stored carbohydrate requires three grams of water to be stored with it. (TRUE)

19. Pregnant women should increase their caloric intake by about 300 calories. (FALSE)

20. To gain muscle weight, consume a higher percentage of protein. (FALSE)

Essay Questions

1. Discuss the reasons behind Americans' obsession with dieting.

2. Describe the energy balance and set point theories of weight control.

3. Identify three factors that influence metabolic rate.

4. Identify and discuss three factors that influence the amount of body fat a person has.

5. Discuss some of the reasons people develop eating disorders.

6. Describe the role of exercise in weight-loss.

7. Identify three ways to decrease fat intake.

8. Explain common traits (claims) which make up a fad or improper diet.

9. Identify three weight-loss myths.

10. Explain who might want to gain weight and how it should be done.

11. Explain how to maintain a healthy percentage of body fat.

Multiple Choice

1. Cardiovascular disease is the number _____ cause of death among American adults.
   a. one
   b. two
   c. three
   d. four

   answer: A(1)

2. Cardiovascular disease starts:
   a. early in life
   b. in the 30's
   c. in the 40's
   d. in the 50's

   answer: A(2)

3. Which of the following is NOT a risk factor for cardiovascular disease?
   a. chronic stress
   b. obesity
   c. sexually transmitted diseases
   d. age

   answer: C(1)

4. Which of the following is NOT one of the modifiable risk factors for heart disease?
   a. smoking
   b. heredity
   c. inactivity
   d. hypertension

   answer: B(2)

5. The prevalence of heart disease has _____ since the 1950's.
   a. increased slightly
   b. increased two-fold
   c. plateaued
   d. decreased by 50 percent

   answer: D(2)

6. Much of the incidence of cardiovascular disease is due to:
   a. an individual's lifestyle
   b. exposure to pollutants
   c. infections
   d. the overuse of antibiotics

   answer: A(2)

7. Which of the following is NOT a common CVD?
   a. stroke
   b. cancer
   c. hypertension
   d. coronary heart disease

   answer: B(1)

8. Any arterial disease that leads to thickening and hardening of the arteries is called:
   a. arteriosclerosis
   b. arthritis
   c. angioplasty
   d. angina pectoris

   answer: A(1)

9. Which of the following is NOT related to a lack of oxygen?
   a. angina pectoris
   b. ischemia
   c. hypoglycemia
   d. myocardial infarction

   answer: C(3)

10. A heart attack is caused by:
    a. a blocked cerebral artery
    b. a blocked coronary artery
    c. a blockage in any main artery in the body
    d. all of the above

    answer: B(3)

11. A stroke is caused by:
    a. a lack of oxygen to the brain
    b. an aneurysm in the brain
    c. a thrombosis blocking a cerebral artery
    d. all of the above

    answer: D(2)

12. Which of the following is NOT a symptom of stroke?
    a. sudden weakness on one side of the face, arm, or leg
    b. slurring of speech
    c. tightening of the chest
    d. unexplained dizziness

    answer: C(2)

13. Which of the following is NOT a warning sign for a heart attack?
    a. small seizures
    b. shortness of breath
    c. pain that spreads to the shoulder, neck, or arm
    d. uncomfortable pressure or pain of the chest

    answer: A(2)

14. Smoking causes an increase in CVD risk for all of the following reasons EXCEPT:
    a. nicotine negatively affects blood cholesterol
    b. nicotine causes the heart rate to decrease to moderately dangerous levels
    c. some of the oxygen flow to the arteries is replaced with carbon monoxide
    d. blood vessels constrict causing blood pressure to increase

    answer: B(3)

15. Factors linked to high blood pressure include:
    a. age, obesity, inactivity
    b. heredity, race, stress
    c. excessive alcohol consumption, sodium sensitivity
    d. all of the above

    answer: D(1)

16. Blood pressure is considered hypertensive when it is consistently above _____ mm of mercury:
    a. 110/75
    b. 120/80
    c. 130/85
    d. 140/90

    answer: D(1)

17. The numerator in the blood pressure fraction represents the _____ pressure.
    a. arterial
    b. diastolic
    c. systolic
    d. valsalvic

    answer: C(1)

18. Heart disease risk is lowest when a person has:
    a. low HDL, and low LDL levels
    b. low HDL, and high LDL levels
    c. high HDL, and low LDL levels
    d. high HDL, and high LDL levels

    answer: C(2)

19. Cholesterol does NOT help:
    a. build cell membranes
    b. control blood sugar levels
    c. digest fat
    d. produce sex characteristic hormones

    answer: B(2)

20. Which of the following can increase the level of HDLs?
    a. steroid use
    b. diabetes
    c. regular exercise
    d. all of the above

    answer: C(1)

21. LDLs can be reduced by eating a diet:
    a. low in saturated fats
    b. high in protein
    c. low in fiber
    d. all of the above

    answer: A(2)

22. Total cholesterol below _____ mg/dl is desirable:
    a. 100
    b. 200
    c. 250
    d. 300

    answer: B(1)

23. Cholesterol:
    a. is found in animal foods
    b. is produced by the liver
    c. is produced to a greater extent when saturated fat is available
    d. all of the above

    answer: D(2)

24. Prolonged high blood pressure can:
    a. cause arteries to become hard and rigid
    b. enlarge the heart muscle
    c. lead to kidney, liver, and eye damage
    d. all of the above

    answer: D(2)

25. Blood pressure can be reduced by:
    a. increasing sodium intake
    b. drinking 3–4 alcoholic drinks per day
    c. losing excess fat
    d. all of the above

    answer: C(2)

26. Blood pressure:
    a. increases during exercise
    b. lowers below pre-exercise levels following exercise
    c. lowers over time with regular exercise
    d. all of the above

    answer: D(2)

27. Which of the following statements is FALSE?
    a. younger women have a lower risk of cardiovascular disease than men
    b. younger people have a lower risk of cardiovascular disease than older people
    c. Caucasian American males have a higher risk than African American males
    d. all of the above

    answer: C(2)

28. Which of the following tests uses sound waves to create a 3-D picture of the heart?
    a. EKG
    b. thallium test
    c. echocardiogram
    d. x-ray

    answer: C(1)

238

29. Which of the following involves the surgical
attachment of a leg vein to the aorta and
blocked artery below the blockage?
    a. coronary artery by-pass
    b. balloon angioplasty
    c. anti-clotting drugs
    d. heart transplant

    answer: A(2)

True/False

1. Cardiovascular disease is the number one killer of American adults. (TRUE)

2. Cardiovascular disease is responsible for almost one half of all adult deaths. (TRUE)

3. The prevalence of heart disease has doubled in the last decade. (FALSE)

4. Lifestyle changes and improved medical treatments are largely responsible for the decrease in the number of cases of heart disease. (TRUE)

5. Atherosclerosis is a cardiovascular disease in which plaque formation narrows the arteries. (TRUE)

6. Atherosclerosis doesn't begin to develop until late in life. (FALSE)

7. The most common risk factor for stroke is hypertension. (TRUE)

8. A stroke is caused by a blockage of a coronary artery. (FALSE)

9. Drugs that can dissolve blood clots in the arteries of heart attack and stroke victims must be taken within 3–6 hours. (TRUE)

10. High cholesterol is often referred to as the "silent killer." (FALSE)

11. Regular exercise can help reduce more than one risk factor for heart disease. (TRUE)

12. Cholesterol is a by-product of metabolism and has no functional use. (FALSE)

13. HDL is called the "good cholesterol" because it helps move cholesterol out of the blood. (TRUE)

14. LDL releases cholesterol to body cells including blood vessel walls. (TRUE)

15. For every one percent decrease in cholesterol, there is a corresponding two percent decrease in heart disease risk. (TRUE)

16. Total cholesterol above 200 mg/dl is desirable. (FALSE)

17. Once you have cardiovascular disease, there is little you can do to reverse the process. (FALSE)

18. A diet high in fiber and low in fat (especially saturated fat) is recommended to reduce cholesterol. (TRUE)

19. A diet high in complex carbohydrates and low in fat is recommended for reducing a person's risk of cardiovascular disease. (TRUE)

Short Answer/Essay

1. Name three of the most common cardiovascular diseases.

2. What is the trend for incidence of cardiovascular disease? Why?

3. Explain the relationship of lifestyle habits and cardiovascular disease.

4. Explain how arteriosclerosis develops and what causes it.

5. What are the signs of a heart attack? stroke? hypertension?

6. What are the modifiable and nonmodifiable risk factors for cardiovascular disease?

7. What impact does regular exercise have on cardiovascular disease?

8. What are the sources of cholesterol, and how can individuals control their cholesterol level?

9. Explain "good" and "bad" cholesterol.

10. What are the dangers of high blood pressure?

11. How can blood pressure be controlled?

12. Can cardiovascular disease be reversed, and if so, how?

13. How is heart disease diagnosed?

14. How is heart disease treated?

Multiple Choice

1. Cancer
   a. is the number two cause of death
   b. is responsible for one out of two deaths in the U.S.
   c. is on the rise
   d. all of the above

   answer: A(1)

2. Which of the following types of cancer are the most common?
   a. bladder, kidney, stomach
   b. prostate, lung, colon and rectal
   c. esophagus, stomach, liver
   d. melanoma of the skin, kidney, leukemia

   answer: B(1)

3. Cancer is characterized by
   a. fever and cramps
   b. an uncontrolled growth of abnormal cells
   c. the development of benign tumors
   d. constriction of the blood vessels leading to the heart

   answer: B(2)

4. Tumors are
   a. foreign bodies lodged in natural tissue
   b. the bulbous ends of plants that when eaten help prevent cancer
   c. abnormal clusters of cells
   d. the result of internal bleeding

   answer: C(2)

5. Some types of cancer can spread
   a. to adjacent tissues
   b. through the bloodstream
   c. through the lymphatic system
   d. all of the above

   answer: D(2)

6. When cancer spreads, it is said to have
   a. enlarged
   b. cloned
   c. augmented
   d. metastasized

   answer: D(1)

7. Which of the following statements is FALSE?
   a. Benign tumors are mildly cancerous.
   b. Benign tumors become dangerous if they crowd other tissues and interrupt normal function.
   c. Malignant tumors can appear in different places in the body at the same time.
   d. Malignant tumors are life threatening.

   answer: A(3)

8. To determine if a cell is cancerous it must be:
   a. examined under a microscope
   b. screened through a blood test
   c. tagged with a radioisotope and x-rayed
   d. none of the above

   answer: A(3)

9. Which of the following is NOT a theory supported by experts and research about how cancer develops?
   a. cancer is the result of a spontaneous error that occurs during cell reproduction
   b. genetic errors that result in cancer sometimes occur when cells are older, or subjected to extreme stress or injury
   c. exposure to certain cancer-causing substances kills cells and stops tissue growth
   d. gene sequences called oncogenes activate and interrupt normal cell reproduction

   answer: C(3)

10. All of the following are considered carcinogens EXCEPT?
    a. tar from cigarette smoke
    b. sodium
    c. ultraviolet light
    d. excessive alcohol

    answer: B(1)

11. Cancer risk is highest among:
    a. Caucasian women
    b. African American men
    c. Native American men
    d. Hispanic women

    answer: B(1)

12. Which of the following substances is a cancer-causing agent found at worksites?
    a. asbestos
    b. inhalants and solvents for painting and auto repair
    c. herbicides and pesticides used in farming
    d. all of the above

    answer: D(1)

13. There is some evidence linking nitrates to:
    a. lung cancer
    b. stomach and esophageal cancer
    c. leukemia
    d. breast cancer

    answer: B(2)

14. The artificial sweetener saccharin:
    a. has the backing of the American Diabetes Association
    b. has been found to be cancer-causing to human beings
    c. has been found to be cancer-causing in high doses in animal studies
    d. all of the above

    answer: D(2)

15. The number one cause of cancer is:
    a. cigarette smoke
    b. ultraviolet light
    c. high fat foods
    d. radiation

    answer: A(1)

16. Which of the following is NOT true about tobacco and cancer?
    a. Pregnant women who smoke risk getting cancer but there is no danger to the fetus.
    b. People who smoke two or more packs a day are more likely to die of cancer.
    c. Breathing second hand smoke can increase lung cancer risk three-fold.
    d. Pipe smoking increases the risk of developing mouth and throat cancer.

    answer: A(3)

17. Which of the following types of cancer is the most common and accounts for the most deaths?
    a. carcinomas
    b. sarcomas
    c. lymphomas
    d. leukemia

    answer: A(2)

18. Which of the following types of cancer occurs in blood-forming parts of the body?
    a. carcinomas
    b. sarcomas
    c. leukemia
    d. lymphomas

    answer: C(2)

19. Smokers reduce their risk of lung cancer to that of a non-smoker after being smoke-free for:
    a. 3 years
    b. 5 years
    c. 10 years
    d. 12 years

    answer: C(1)

20. The lowest survival rate of cancer occurs with which of the following types of cancer?
    a. lung
    b. breast
    c. skin
    d. colon

    answer: A(2)

21. Which of the following is NOT a risk factor for breast cancer?
    a. amount of breast tissue
    b. alcohol, 3 drinks a week
    c. family history
    d. never having a child

    answer: A(2)

22. Which of the following does NOT increase a women's risk of breast cancer?
    a. early menarche
    b. late menopause
    c. obesity
    d. hormone replacement therapy

    answer: D(2)

23. A screening test for breast cancer is called a:
    a. Pap test
    b. mammogram
    c. MRI
    d. CAT scan

    answer: B(1)

24. Treatments for breast cancer include:
    a. lumpectomy
    b. radical mastectomy
    c. radiation therapy
    d. all of the above

    answer: D(2)

25. Risk of skin cancer increases with all of the following EXCEPT:
    a. family history
    b. working in a dark, damp environment
    c. red or blond hair
    d. three or more severe sunburns as a teenager

    answer: B(2)

26. Seventy five percent of lung cancer is related to:
    a. smoking
    b. poor diet
    c. asbestos
    d. second-hand smoke

    answer: A(1)

27. The overall number of cancer cases is dropping, but one type is increasing. It is:
    a. colon and rectal cancer
    b. breast cancer
    c. Hodgkin's disease
    d. leukemia

    answer: B(1)

28. A major risk factor for colon and rectal cancer is a:
    a. high fat diet
    b. diet low in fiber
    c. sedentary lifestyle
    d. all of the above

    answer: D(2)

29. A history of multiple sex partners and STDs puts a man at increased risk for:
    a. prostate cancer
    b. colon and rectal cancer
    c. throat cancer
    d. breast cancer

    answer: A(2)

30. Cancer risk can be lowered by:
    a. eating foods high in antioxidants
    b. drinking a glass of wine a day
    c. grilling food rather than broiling it
    d. drinking a glass of milk daily

    answer: A(2)

31. Which of the following statements is FALSE?
    a. sedentary individuals have a 30–100 percent higher risk of cancer
    b. poorly fit individuals have higher risk than moderately fit individuals
    c. exercise must be vigorous to lower cancer risk
    d. women who are fit have a lower incidence of breast and reproductive organ cancer

    answer: C(2)

32. Cancer can be treated using all of the following EXCEPT:
    a. chemotherapy
    b. radiation therapy
    c. psychotherapy
    d. immunotherapy

    answer: C(1)

33. Cancers can be detected using all of the following EXCEPT:
    a. biopsy
    b. cell mapping
    c. MRI
    d. CAT scan

    answer: B(1)

34. Diabetes is a:
    a. metabolic disease
    b. nervous disorder
    c. cardiorespiratory disease
    d. lymphatic disease

    answer: A(1)

35. A severe allergic response can result in:
    a. a diabetic coma
    b. heat exhaustion
    c. anaphylactic shock
    d. a stroke

    answer: C(1)

36. Psychological headaches are caused by:
    a. the side effects of some other underlying cause
    b. the rapid constriction and dilation of blood vessels
    c. involuntary muscle tension
    d. anxiety, depression, mental and emotional stress

    answer: D(2)

True/False

1. Socioeconomic conditions and reduced access to treatment may account for lower cancer survival rates among African Americans as compared to Caucasians. (TRUE)

2. Lung, colon and rectal, and breast cancer account for over half of all cancer cases. (TRUE)

3. A tumor is by definition malignant. (FALSE)

4. Cancer is one disease. (FALSE)

5. Persons who have inherited oncogenes will eventually develop cancer. (FALSE)

6. Carcinogens are those substances or environmental agents that are believed to be related to cancer. (TRUE)

7. African American males have a higher death rate from cancer than other races. (TRUE)

8. Different types of cancer occur with the same frequency in both men and women. (FALSE)

9. All artificial sweeteners have been proven to cause cancer in humans. (FALSE)

10. The more estrogen in a women's body over her lifetime, the greater her risk of breast cancer. (TRUE)

11. The five year survival rate for breast cancer has increased from 78% in 1940 to 92% today. (TRUE)

12. The most common types of skin cancers affect the squamous and basal layers of the skin and usually don't spread. (TRUE)

13. A cancer diagnosis is a death sentence. (FALSE)

14. Type I, insulin dependent diabetes accounts for 90 percent of diabetes. (FALSE)

15. The number of people with asthma is increasing. (TRUE)

16. People with asthma or diabetes should avoid cardiorespiratory endurance exercise. (FALSE)

17. Diabetes is strictly an adult disease. (FALSE)

18. Allergies can be inherited. (TRUE)

19. The allergic response is an over reaction of a person's own immune system. (TRUE)

20. Tension headaches are more common than secondary or migraine headaches. (TRUE)

Short Answer/Essay

1. Identify four lifestyle habits that can reduce a person's risk of cancer.

2. Name the three most common cancers for men and the three most common for women.

3. Describe the four kinds of cancer.

4. Explain how cancer spreads.

5. Discuss the theories of how cancer develops.

6. Select one kind of cancer and explain how to prevent, detect, and treat it.

7. Explain the role of exercise in the management of asthma and diabetes.

8. Describe the four types of headaches.

9. List five common allergens.

Multiple Choice

1. Stress arises from:
   a. something external to the person that causes mental and/or physical tension
   b. an internal state of a person
   c. from a transaction between a person and the environment
   d. all of the above

   answer: D(2)

2. Too little stress is called:
   a. hypostress
   b. eustress
   c. distress
   d. mistress

   answer: A(1)

3. Which of the following is an example of eustress?
   a. an automobile accident
   b. graduation nerves
   c. test anxiety
   d. illness

   answer: B(2)

4. Which of the following is an example of hypostress?
   a. an elderly person who lives alone and has nothing to do
   b. a retired person who volunteers in the schools
   c. a young person going to school and working
   d. a middle-aged person working 70-hour weeks

   answer: A(2)

5. The stress associated with making a decision about what is right and wrong is:
   a. emotional stress
   b. spiritual stress
   c. physical stress
   d. mental stress

   answer: B(2)

6. To maintain a healthy mental outlook:
   a. seek out challenging mental activities
   b. seek out relaxing activities
   c. look at change as something normal
   d. all of the above

   answer: D(2)

7. Which of the following is associated with stress-related disease?
   a. eustress
   b. distress
   c. homeostasis
   d. arousal

   answer: B(2)

8. To reduce your risk of stress-related disease, you should try to:
   a. control your hostility and anger
   b. control how you perceive and react to stress
   c. limit your contact with stressors you can avoid
   d. all of the above

   answer: D(2)

9. The inverted "U" hypothesis describes the relationship between:
   a. arousal, stress and performance
   b. alarm, resistance and exhaustion
   c. eustress, distress and homeostasis
   d. none of the above

   answer: A(2)

10. Stress is studied from which perspective?
    a. physical reactions
    b. mental and emotional reactions
    c. reactions to social pressures
    d. all of the above

    answer: D(1)

11. Homeostasis is:
    a. a tendency of an organism to maintain a stable internal environment
    b. a body's internal response to acute stress
    c. the breakdown of biological systems
    d. an environmental condition leading to stress

    answer: A(1)

12. Common physiological responses to stress are:
    a. a decrease in body temperature and mobility
    b. elevated heart rate and body temperature
    c. rapid eye movement
    d. a loss of hand-eye coordination

    answer: B(2)

13. Selye identified a 3-stage stress response called the General Adaptation Syndrome. The correct order for the three stages is:
    a. alarm, resistance, exhaustion.
    b. resistance, alarm, exhaustion.
    c. exhaustion, alarm, resistance
    d. alarm, exhaustion, resistance

    answer: A(1)

14. The alarm response is characterized by an:
    a. increase in alertness and muscle tension
    b. decrease in motor skill
    c. increase in urine production and decrease in sweating
    d. increase in blood flow to surface vessels thereby flushing the face and skin

    answer: A(2)

15. The exhaustion stage occurs when what is depleted?
    a. your will to resist
    b. your calorie intake for that day
    c. your adaptive energy reserve
    d. your adrenaline reserve

    answer: C(2)

16. Which of the following is an example of social/environmental stress?
    a. test anxiety
    b. construction noise
    c. unexpected expense
    d. all of the above

    answer: B(2)

17. In Lazarus' Cognitive Transitional Model, demands are determined by:
    a. individual perceptions
    b. absolute values
    c. group study
    d. peer pressure

    answer: A(2)

18. Which of these is not a cognitive side effect of chronic stress?
    a. emotional outbursts
    b. anger displacement
    c. distorted perception
    d. physical exhaustion

    answer: D(2)

19. According to psychologists, the stress response is dictated by all of the following EXCEPT:
    a. the actual stressor
    b. a person's perception of the stressor
    c. a person's ability to meet the demands of the stressor
    d. a person's personality type

    answer: A(2)

20. Which personality type is the most stress resistant?
    a. Type A
    b. Type B
    c. Type C
    d. Type E

    answer: C(2)

21. Which of the following is not a good stress survival tool?
    a. identifying the stressors in your life
    b. taking control when you can
    c. accepting your limitations
    d. drinking alcohol to relax

    answer: D(2)

22. Which of the following cognitive interventions may distort the truth?
    a. reframing
    b. rationalizing
    c. imagery
    d. positive self-talk

    answer: B(2)

23. When using imagery you should try to use which of your senses?
    a. sight and hearing
    b. sight and touch
    c. smell and touch
    d. all five senses

    answer: D(2)

24. Good time management does not include:
    a. prioritizing tasks
    b. setting aside personal work time
    c. saving the most difficult task for last
    d. learning to say no

    answer: C(2)

25. Which of the following is NOT a relaxation technique?
    a. autogenic training
    b. transcendental meditation
    c. biofeedback
    d. homeostatic conditioning

    answer: D(2)

26. Progressive relaxation is:
    a. a physiological technique
    b. a cognitive technique
    c. a time management technique
    d. impossible for type A people to master

    answer: A(2)

27. Autogenic means:
    a. produced independently of external influence or aid
    b. produced by external influence
    c. produced by chemical reaction
    d. none of the above

    answer: A(2)

28. A mantra is associated with:
    a. progressive relaxation
    b. autogenic training
    c. meditation
    d. biofeedback

    answer: C(2)

29. Biofeedback techniques teach you how to exert voluntary control over certain functions of the:
    a. autonomic nervous system
    b. gastronomic system
    c. skeletal system
    d. none of the above

    answer: A(2)

30. Mood rings function under the principles of
    a. biofeedback
    b. transcendental meditation
    c. rationalization
    d. social stress

    answer: A(1)

31. Laughter:
    a. diffuses physical tension and triggers a relaxation response
    b. causes physical tension
    c. is part of meditation training
    d. none of the above

    answer: A(2)

32. Which of the following names is NOT associated with stress research?
    a. Hans Selye
    b. Susanne Kobasa
    c. Richard Lazarus
    d. Steven Blair

    answer: D(2)

True/False

1. Physiologists and psychologists agree on how to define and explain stress. (FALSE)

2. Too much stress is called hypostress. (FALSE)

3. A high percentage of doctor visits are the result of stress-related illness. (TRUE)

4. A lack of social interaction can be as harmful as negative social relationships. (TRUE)

5. Stress does not occur when the stressor is imagined. (FALSE)

6. If a person believes that a situation will result in loss, harm or threat, the person will experience stress. (TRUE)

7. The resistance stage is reached when chronic stress forces the body to establish a new level of homeostasis. (TRUE)

8. Daily hassles and small irritating problems may be more significant to health risk than major life stressors. (TRUE)

9. The perception of the stressor is sometimes more problematic than the stressor. (TRUE)

10. Too little stress can be as detrimental to performance as too much stress. (TRUE)

11. Relaxation techniques can be mastered in a few days. (FALSE)

12. Cognitive intervention strategies mainly target problems of a physical origin. (FALSE)

13. Burnout is an example of physical stress. (FALSE)

14. Fight or flight was first described by Walter Cannon. (TRUE)

15. Hans Selye is considered the pioneer of stress research. (TRUE)

16. The general adaptation syndrome describes a person's mental response to stress. (FALSE)

17. Persons with Type B personalities are more prone to heart disease. (FALSE)

18. Life requires stress. (TRUE)

Short Answer/Essay

1. Define stress.

2. Differentiate between and give examples of distress, eustress, and hypostress.

3. Provide two examples each of physical, social, mental, and spiritual stress.

4. Give examples of how too much and too little physical, mental, social and spiritual stress can be detrimental.

5. Describe the different approaches to stress research of biologists/physiologists, psychologists and sociologists.

6. Describe the general adaptation syndrome (G.A.S.).

7. How does personality interact with stress?

8. How are hardy people different from others?

9. Discuss life event changes and daily hassles as they relate to stress.

10. What does it mean to take an interdisciplinary approach to stress?

11. What is the difference between a cognitive intervention and a physiological one?

12. Describe three cognitive interventions.

13. Describe three physiological interventions.

14. Name five ways to improve time management.

15. Provide three examples of how you can reduce stress in your life.

Creating and Maintaining Healthy Relationships

Multiple Choice

1. Which of the following describes an intimate relationship?
   a. two people sharing their experiences as abused children
   b. two people sharing a monogamous sexual relationship
   c. two people working together for years to achieve a shared purpose
   d. all of the above

   answer: D(2)

2. The lack of healthy relationships in one's life can result in:
   a. isolation and loneliness
   b. intellectual freedom
   c. social freedom
   d. all of the above

   answer: A(2)

3. The three stages of maturity are:
   a. me, you, us
   b. the individual, the family, the community
   c. selfishness, learned tolerance, selflessness
   d. being human-centered, community-centered, world-centered

   answer: C(1)

4. Being able to accept that you will not always get what you want demonstrates:
   a. sharing
   b. obedience
   c. selflessness
   d. learned tolerance

   answer: D(2)

5. Selflessness:
   a. is the ability to put someone else first
   b. means to lose one's own identity
   c. is thinking only of one's own needs
   d. is a natural part of a young person's life

   answer: A(2)

6. Which of the following describes learned tolerance?
   a. taking your paycheck and buying something you've always wanted
   b. shoveling the sidewalk for a relative without being asked
   c. meeting a midnight curfew even though you don't believe it matters
   d. all of the above

   answer: C(3)

7. Which of the following describes selflessness?
   a. a young child placing his full trust in a parent
   b. a person abstaining from sexual intercourse until his/her partner is ready
   c. driving the speed limit even when no one is out on the streets
   d. all of the above

   answer: B(3)

8. Men and women often express friendship differently. Which of the following is more typical of men?
    a. to do things together rather than talk
    b. to talk and listen using expressive communication
    c. to use touch such as hugs
    d. to offer verbal support and understanding

    answer: A(2)

9. Which of the following is LEAST likely to nurture a friendship?
    a. confiding in a friend
    b. spending time together
    c. giving a friend advice on how to become a better person
    d. a willingness to share material things

    answer: C(2)

10. Dating is a good opportunity to:
    a. learn more about the other person
    b. meet new people
    c. see if there is more than a physical attraction
    d. all of the above

    answer: D(2)

11. Happily married people:
    a. live longer than unmarried people
    b. have a legal and financial advantage over single people
    c. have a lower risk of sexually transmitted diseases
    d. all of the above

    answer: D(2)

12. Which of the following statements is FALSE?
    a. about 50 percent of American families are traditional families (working father, homemaker mother, children)
    b. single parent families are on the rise
    c. since 1960 the number of births to unwed parents and teen parents has quadrupled
    d. more than 50 percent of children can expect to spend at least one year living in a single-parent home before the age of 18

    answer: A(3)

13. Which of the following is NOT part of the predictable cycle of events in family violence?
    a. avoidance so as not to provoke the other person
    b. accumulated grievances which erupt into violence
    c. period where grievances are outwardly expressed toward a third party
    d. a period of conciliation and remorse

    answer: C(3)

14. Poor relationships may suffer from:
    a. poor communication
    b. lack of time spent together
    c. physical, sexual or emotional abuse
    d. all of the above

    answer: D(1)

15. Which of the following is NOT a reason that the number of people living single is increasing?
    a. an increasing number of people who are divorced
    b. elderly women outliving their husbands
    c. more people preferring not to marry
    d. people staying single longer before marrying

    answer: C(2)

True/False

1. An intimate relationship by definition includes physical intimacy. (FALSE)

2. Teenagers who have learned to follow rules even if they don't fully understand the purpose of the rule have acquired learned tolerance. (TRUE)

3. Everyone eventually grows out of the selfishness stage. (FALSE)

4. Supportive friends and family help buffer against stress-related illness. (TRUE)

5. Most long-term friendships are formed in adolescence. (TRUE)

6. Lasting relationships are characterized by unconditional love. (TRUE)

7. Married men are more prone to alcoholism. (FALSE)

8. High blood pressure, hormone changes, and the stress response can result from problems in an unhappy marriage. (TRUE)

9. There is no such thing as fair fighting. (FALSE)

10. For a marriage to succeed, both individuals need to have realistic expectations about each other. (TRUE)

11. The vast majority of people want to get married. (TRUE)

12. A traditional family is defined as one with two working parents. (FALSE)

13. Family structure has changed over the past few decades. (TRUE)

14. Counseling is a viable alternative for a relationship in trouble. (TRUE)

15. Family violence occurs across all segments of society. (TRUE)

16. Family violence can be physical or psychological. (TRUE)

17. Children from abusive families are less likely to be abusive themselves. (FALSE)

18. A relationship should be terminated when it is abusive. (TRUE)

19. Research shows a strong correlation between loneliness and premature death and illness. (TRUE)

20. Loneliness can be cured by building social contacts and support. (TRUE)

21. Healthy relationships support emotional, mental, social, and physical wellness. (TRUE)

Short Answer/Essay

1. Discuss how healthy relationships influence the dimensions of wellness.

2. Name, describe, and give an example for each of the three stages of maturity.

3. Define an intimate relationship.

4. Give some suggestions for how to nurture a friendship.

5. Give some examples of things that tend to keep a marriage healthy.

6. Describe some of the signs of an unhealthy relationship.

7. Discuss how and why the family structure has changed in the last few decades.

8. Explain who is single and why the number of single people is increasing.

9. What are the effects of loneliness, and how can it be cured?

Multiple Choice

1. Which age group accounts for the highest number of cases of STDs?
   a. 15–29 years
   b. 20–35 years
   c. 25–39 years
   d. 35–45 years

   answer: A(1)

2. STDs can NOT be caused by:
   a. viruses
   b. fungus
   c. bacteria
   d. cancer

   answer: D(1)

3. People with STDs can transmit the disease:
   a. when they are asymptomatic or symptomatic
   b. only when they are symptomatic
   c. only during a four-week window following infection
   d. only when their partner has a weakened immune system

   answer: A(2)

4. STD infections can lead to:
   a. pelvic inflammatory disease
   b. cancer
   c. sterility
   d. all of the above

   answer: D(2)

5. Before having sexual intercourse, partners should:
   a. talk to one another about their sexual histories
   b. have a medical check-up
   c. look for outward signs of disease
   d. all of the above

   answer: D(1)

6. Who is at the LEAST risk for STD infection ?
   a. homosexual men
   b. homosexual women
   c. heterosexual women
   d. heterosexual men

   answer: B(3)

7. Which of the following behaviors carries the greatest risk?
   a. receptive vaginal intercourse
   b. oral sex on a man with ejaculation
   c. oral sex on a woman
   d. intimate kissing

   answer: A(2)

8. When symptoms appear, they typically include:
   a. burning or pain during urination or defecation
   b. itching or burning around the genitals
   c. mucus discharge or bleeding from the genitals
   d. all of the above

   answer: D(2)

9. Women are less likely than men to seek treatment because they:
   a. are asymptomatic more often than men
   b. take their health less seriously than men
   c. are more embarrassed than men
   d. blame symptoms on their menstrual cycle

   answer: A(2)

10. HIV does all of the following EXCEPT:
    a. weakens the immune system
    b. kills T-cells
    c. is associated with an unexplained weight gain
    d. opens the door to other infections

    answer: C(2)

11. HIV can NOT be transmitted:
    a. through casual kissing
    b. through needle sharing
    c. through unprotected sex
    d. from a mother to an unborn child

    answer: A(1)

12. HIV can be transmitted:
    a. through wound to wound contact with an infected person.
    b. through a bite from an infected mosquito.
    c. by sharing a cup used by an infected person.
    d. all of the above

    answer: A(2)

13. AIDS was first discovered in the United States in:
    a. 1964
    b. 1972
    c. 1978
    d. 1985

    answer: C(1)

14. Which of the following is NOT an early symptom of HIV infection?
    a. swollen glands
    b. night sweats
    c. genital warts
    d. weight loss

    answer: C(1)

15. It takes _____ following HIV infection for the body to produce enough antibodies to be detected by a blood test.
    a. 1–3 weeks
    b. 1–2 months
    c. 3–6 months
    d. 1–2 years

    answer: C(1)

16. Which of the following forms of hepatitis is most often transmitted sexually?
    a. hepatitis A
    b. hepatitis B
    c. hepatitis C
    d. all of the above

    answer: B(1)

17. Prevention for hepatitis B includes all of the following EXCEPT:
    a. avoiding contaminated needles
    b. getting vaccinated
    c. practicing safe sex or abstinence
    d. avoiding contaminated drinking water

    answer: D(2)

18. Of the following which is the LEAST common STD?
    a. gonorrhea
    b. chlamydia
    c. human papillomavirus (HPV)
    d. syphilis

    answer: D(2)

19. Which statement about gonorrhea is FALSE?
    a. Men are more easily infected than women.
    b. Eighty percent of women who are infected will not have symptoms.
    c. It is the most common cause of pelvic inflammatory disease (PID).
    d. If it spreads to the bloodstream, it can affect the heart, spinal cord, or brain.

    answer: A(2)

20. Which of the following diseases can cause blindness in a newborn if left untreated?
    a. gonorrhea
    b. syphilis
    c. chlamydia
    d. trichomoniasis

    answer: A(2)

21. Pelvic inflammatory disease (PID):
    a. is a bone disease associated with STDs.
    b. occurs when infectious bacteria escape into the pelvic cavity.
    c. is the result of abnormal menstruation.
    d. is caused by the AIDS virus.

    answer: B(2)

22. Which of the following is NOT true of pelvic inflammatory disease (PID)?
    a. women over age 25 are at more risk than younger women
    b. it can cause sterility
    c. it increases the risk of an ectopic pregnancy
    d. it can cause chronic pelvic pain

    answer: A(2)

23. Which of the following diseases can lie dormant for as many as 40 years?
    a. chlamydia
    b. HIV
    c. syphilis
    d. all of the above

    answer: D(2)

24. Which of the following diseases is caused by a virus?
    a. syphilis
    b. hepatitis B
    c. gonorrhea
    d. genital herpes

    answer: D(1)

25. A chancre develops at the entry site for which disease?
    a. syphilis
    b. hepatitis B
    c. chlamydia
    d. HIV

    answer: A(2)

26. A body rash, open sores around the genitals and mouth, and swollen lymph nodes are signs of _____ syphilis.
    a. primary
    b. secondary
    c. latent
    d. tertiary

    answer: B(2)

27. If left untreated, syphilis can result in:
    a. impaired hearing and vision
    b. memory loss and depression
    c. heart disease and paralysis
    d. all of the above

    answer: D(2)

28. The "silent STD" is the nickname given to _____ because its early symptoms are so mild.
    a. HPV
    b. syphilis
    c. chlamydia
    d. genital herpes

    answer: C(2)

29. Antibiotics are an effective treatment for:
    a. HIV
    b. genital herpes
    c. chlamydia
    d. HPV

    answer: C(1)

30. Which two diseases are very similar and together account for most of the cases of PID?
    a. genital herpes and hepatitis B
    b. chlamydia and gonorrhea
    c. HIV and AIDS
    d. candidiasis and trichomoniasis

    answer: B(1)

31. Genital herpes is all of the following EXCEPT:
    a. caused by the herpes simplex virus (HSV-2)
    b. a painful disease that causes painful blisters on genitals, mouth, and anus
    c. an infection that can cause blindness and brain damage to babies
    d. an infection that men get four times more easily from women than women get it from men

    answer: D(2)

32. In which disease does the virus travel on the sensory nerve and settle in the ganglia near the spinal cord and then periodically travel back down the nerve and multiply near the skin again?
    a. genital herpes
    b. syphilis
    c. HIV
    d. gonorrhea

    answer: A(1)

33. Which of the following is a fungal disease?
    a. trichomoniasis
    b. candidiasis
    c. pubic lice
    d. HPV

    answer: B(1)

34. Which disease is detected in women using a Pap smear?
    a. trichomoniasis
    b. genital herpes
    c. HIV
    d. HPV

    answer: D(2)

35. Which disease can you get from infected clothing, sheets, towels, or a toilet seat?
    a. pubic lice
    b. HIV
    c. syphilis
    d. all of the above

    answer: A(1)

36. Which of the following is NOT true concerning HPV?
    a. compared to other STDs, sexual transmission of HPV is infrequent
    b. some forms of the disease are linked to cancer
    c. there are over 60 forms of the disease
    d. genital warts appear with some forms of HPV

    answer: A(2)

37. A yeast infection is a form of:
    a. candidiasis
    b. human papillomavirus
    c. trichomoniasis
    d. genital herpes

    answer: A(1)

38. Half of the cases of epididymitis (inflammation of the testicles) is caused by:
    a. HIV
    b. genital herpes
    c. chlamydia
    d. trichomoniasis

    answer: C(2)

39. Which of the following diseases is caused by a protozoan infection?
    a. candidiasis
    b. genital herpes
    c. pubic lice
    d. trichomoniasis

    answer: D(1)

40. Which of the following diseases attacks the liver?
    a. genital herpes
    b. hepatitis B
    c. syphilis
    d. gonorrhea

    answer: B(1)

41. Symptoms of pubic lice include:
    a. pain upon urination
    b. intense itching
    c. vaginal discharge
    d. all of the above

    answer: B(1)

42. Which of the following best describes the relationship between HIV and STDs?
    a. it has no known effect
    b. the suppressive effects of HIV on the immune system worsen the symptoms of STDs and makes them harder to treat
    c. treatments for HIV boost the immune system and make it more difficult to contract other STDs
    d. a person with HIV rarely has another STD so there is too little evidence to establish a relationship between them

    answer: B(3)

43. Which of the following STDs can be contracted through non-sexual means?
    a. HIV
    b. trichomoniasis
    c. pubic lice
    d. all of the above

    answer: D(2)

44. Use of lamb and natural skin condoms is effective:
    a. for birth control
    b. against the AIDS virus
    c. against all STDs except the AIDS virus
    d. none of the above

    answer: A(2)

45. All of the following are good prevention measures against STDs EXCEPT:
    a. abstinence
    b. exclusive sex with a disease-free individual
    c. use of oil-based lubricants with latex condoms
    d. use of a latex condom and a spermicide

    answer: C(2)

260

True/False

1. More than 50 organisms and syndromes are recognized as being involved in STDs. (TRUE)

2. After being infected with an STD, a person may remain asymptomatic for periods ranging from days to months. (TRUE)

3. STD risk is mostly determined by personal behavior, but demographics can play a role. (TRUE)

4. Men are more susceptible to most STDs than women. (FALSE)

5. HIV can be transmitted through food that has been handled by an infected person. (FALSE)

6. AZT treatments during pregnancy can greatly reduce the risk of passing AIDS onto the baby. (TRUE)

7. HIV can be found in blood, semen, vaginal fluids, and breast milk. (TRUE)

8. Blood banks started screening for HIV in 1990. (FALSE)

9. People with HIV who look and feel healthy cannot transmit the disease to someone else. (FALSE)

10. The number of cases of hepatitis B attributed to homosexual contact has dropped, while the portion attributed to heterosexual contact and injection drug use has increased. (TRUE)

11. Men do not get yeast infections. (FALSE)

12. Genital herpes has been linked to cancer. (FALSE)

13. STDs are preventable. (TRUE)

14. The structure of a woman's organs makes her more susceptible to disease than a man. (TRUE)

15. A person in a monogamous relationship with an infected person is at risk during unprotected sex. (TRUE)

16. Gonorrhea can be transmitted through oral sex. (TRUE)

17. Untreated syphilis will often spontaneously clear up. (FALSE)

18. HSV-2 is usually responsible for cold sores. (FALSE)

19. Genital herpes is most likely to be transmitted when one or more partner has open sores. (TRUE)

20. Only a small percentage of HPV cases have visible warts. (TRUE)

21. Trichomoniasis is treated with heat packs because it can't survive in a warm, moist environment. (FALSE)

22. Yeast infections can occur spontaneously without any sexual contact. (TRUE)

23. A person with open sores or warts from one STD is more susceptible to other STDs. (TRUE)

Short Answer/Essay

1. Who is at risk for sexually transmitted disease? Who has the most/least risk?

2. How are STDs transmitted?

3. Discuss the mode of transmission, symptoms, diagnostic tests, and treatment for one STD.

4. Describe five things you can do to diminish or eliminate risk of contracting (or passing on) a sexually transmitted disease.

5. Explain the role of communication in the prevention and management of STDs.

6. Describe high-risk sexual behavior.

7. What types of organisms cause STDs, and how does this influence treatment?

8. Describe the relationship between HIV and other STDs.

9. Name five ways that people mistakenly believe HIV is transmitted. Name three ways that it is transmitted.

10. What are common symptoms for men and women for the most common STDs?

Multiple Choice

1. George's friends throw him a big birthday party, offering him all the alcohol he can drink. Normally not a big drinker, George indulges at the urging of his friends. Driving home from the party, he is in a car wreck and the driver of the other car is killed. This is an example of all of the following EXCEPT:
   a. addiction
   b. substance abuse
   c. social drinking
   d. peer pressure

   answer: A(2)

2. Mary and Beth are student workers at the health center. Mary covers for her friend Beth when she is late to work, sick, or makes mistakes on the job. Beth parties three to four times a week and often cannot remember her own actions from the night before. Which of the following statements is FALSE?
   a. Mary is an enabler.
   b. Beth shows signs of addiction.
   c. Beth is a little irresponsible but with her friends' support she'll get better.
   d. Beth is an example of how substance abuse costs society.

   answer: C(2)

3. Sarah is a popular student at College University. After the homecoming dance and a few beers, she and her boyfriend Tom let their hormones take over. Sarah has learned she is pregnant, and the two of them are dropping out of school to become a family. This is an example of:
   a. a cost to society
   b. addiction
   c. substance abuse
   4. psychological dependence

   answer: A(3)

4. The blood alcohol content (BAC) is affected by all of the following EXCEPT:
   a. drinking coffee
   b. having a full meal with the alcoholic drink
   c. genetic variability of metabolizing enzymes
   d. weight

   answer: A(2)

5. An average woman will experience a greater effect per unit of alcohol than an average man because:
   a. she has a lower percentage of body fat than a man
   b. she has a smaller blood volume than a man
   c. she produces larger amounts of the enzyme alcohol dehydrogenase
   d. she has a higher metabolism

   answer: B(3)

6. Richard is an eight year old who has a reduced ability to learn from experience and who exhibits poor judgment. Richard's mother consumed alcohol while she was pregnant with Richard. Richard's condition is an example of:
    a. fetal alcohol effect
    b. fetal alcohol syndrome
    c. a short term effect that he will outgrow
    d. slow starters

    answer: A(2)

7. All of the following are street names for marijuana EXCEPT:
    a. roach
    b. Mary Jane
    c. toot
    d. grass

    answer: C(1)

8. Which of the following is a powerful hallucinogen?
    a. cocaine
    b. sleeping pills
    c. LSD
    d. marijuana

    answer: C(1)

9. Which of the following is NOT a warning sign of a substance abuse problem?
    a. drinking alone
    b. loss of interest in sex, friends, or hobbies
    c. wide mood swings
    d. occasional incidence of insomnia

    answer: D(2)

10. Children of alcoholic parents are more apt to ____ than other children.
    a. be alcoholics themselves
    b. marry an alcoholic
    c. have an eating disorder
    d. all of the above

    answer: D(2)

11. Alcohol:
    a. depresses the brain center that controls inhibition
    b. elevates serotonin levels in the brain
    c. increases adrenalin, resulting in a surge of energy
    d. stimulates the speech and hearing centers of the brain

    answer: A(2)

12. The most common alcohol-related disease is:
    a. HIV
    b. heart disease
    c. cirrhosis of the liver
    d. cancer

    answer: C(2)

13. Which of the following is NOT an alcohol-related disease?
    a. impotence
    b. diabetes
    c. cancer
    d. heart disease

    answer: B(2)

14. Which of the following is FALSE?
    a. infants can receive alcohol through breast milk
    b. pregnant women who drink risk giving birth to a mentally retarded child
    c. when pregnant, there is no harm in drinking small amounts of alcohol
    d. some women who drink do not know they are pregnant

    answer: C(2)

15. For alcohol and drug treatment to be successful, the program must include:
    a. medical treatment
    b. detoxification
    c. long term behavior change strategies
    d. all of the above

    answer: D(2)

16. The average starting age for smoking cigarettes is _____ years old.
    a. 13
    b. 15
    c. 17
    d. 19

    answer: A(1)

17. In federal buildings it is:
    a. illegal to smoke
    b. legal to smoke
    c. up to the management whether or not smoking is allowed
    d. all of the above

    answer: A(2)

18. What percentage of adults are smokers today?
    a. one quarter
    b. one third
    c. one half
    d. two thirds

    answer: B(2)

True/False

1. Secondhand smoke is classified as either mainstream smoke exhaled from a smoker or sidestream smoke coming directly from a burning cigarette. (TRUE)

2. Working in a smoky bar puts David at a higher risk for lung cancer. (TRUE)

3. A majority of people who go through a medically directed treatment program achieve long term smoking cessation. (FALSE)

4. Marijuana has been used for cancer patients to alleviate nausea and increase appetite. (TRUE)

5. There is no indication of deleterious long term effects of regular long-term use of marijuana. (FALSE)

6. Men report more drinking problems than women. (TRUE)

7. Smoking is the number one cause of lung cancer. (TRUE)

8. After quitting smoking, it usually takes 1-3 weeks before any changes occur. (FALSE)

9. Alcohol absorption is slowed when the stomach is empty. (FALSE)

10. The two most prevalent diseases associated with tobacco use are poor nutrition and cancer.(FALSE)

11. Smokeless tobacco (chew) is not addictive. (FALSE)

Short Answer/Essay

1. How has public opinion concerning tobacco changed in the last 40 years? Include a discussion concerning anti-tobacco legislation.

2. What are the negative consequences of alcohol abuse?

3. Why do people smoke? What benefit do they receive?

4.   What strategies are available to help people quit smoking?

5.   How effective are the various smoking cessation strategies?

6.   What are the documented side effects of marijuana use?

7.   How can alcohol and tobacco use affect unborn children?

8.   How can you talk to a friend or relative about his or her substance abuse problem?

9.   How do you know if you are addicted to something?

10. How does tobacco use kill?

Multiple Choice

1. Change is best accomplished using:
   a. an illness-treatment approach
   b. an all-or-none approach
   c. a one-step-at-a-time approach
   d. all of the above

   answer: C(2)

2. Relapse often occurs when:
   a. other pressing demands occur
   b. you are motivated to change
   c. others support your change
   d. none of the above

   answer: A(2)

3. The human-cultural environment includes all of the following EXCEPT:
   a. people
   b. laws
   c. pets
   d. religious beliefs

   answer: C(1)

4. Which of the following is LEAST likely to be a defining characteristic of a human-cultural environment?
   a. ethnicity
   b. motivation
   c. economic prosperity
   d. age

   answer: B(2)

5. A world view recognizes that:
   a. we are all part of a larger ecosystem
   b. the individual influences world wellness
   c. the environment influences personal wellness
   d. all of the above

   answer: D(2)

6. Which of the following is an example of the individual influencing the human-cultural environment?
   a. a parent cooking well-balanced meals for the family
   b. a student heading up a recycle effort
   c. a support group helping someone cope with a problem
   d. a sorority or fraternity raising money for the American Cancer Society

   answer: A(3)

7. A change in personal behavior can:
   a. be disruptive to others
   b. motivate others to make change
   c. make others uncomfortable
   d. all of the above

   answer: D(2)

8. A human-centered perspective holds that:
    a. the world exists to fulfill human needs
    b. human beings are stewards of the environment
    c. regardless of human usefulness, all environmental resources are valuable
    d. human beings are interdependent with animal and plant life

    answer: A(2)

9. A world-view holds that:
    a. humans dominate the world
    b. everything and everyone is interconnected
    c. human beings are the primary force in changing the environment
    d. the environment will automatically balance human consumption

    answer: C(2)

10. Which of the following is NOT an example of the natural environment influencing the individual?
    a. pollen triggering an asthma attack
    b. garbage strewn along the highway
    c. long dark winter days causing depression
    d. local foods forming the staple of a person's diet

    answer: B(2)

11. Which of the following is an example of the individual influencing the natural environment?
    a. a student throwing a soda can on the ground or in a recycle bin
    b. swimmers getting sick from a bacterial growth in the water
    c. a person suffering altitude sickness during a ski vacation
    d. sunny warm days encouraging physical activity

    answer: A(2)

12. Which of the following statements is FALSE?
    a. people in sunny climates tend to be more physically active
    b. long dark winter days can depress some people
    c. physical exertion on very hot and humid days can be dangerous
    d. exercising at dusk limits exposure to pollens and air pollutants

    answer: D(2)

True/False Questions

1. An illness-treatment approach to change is a short-term fix to a long-term problem. (TRUE)

2. Regression or relapse can happen at any of the five stages of change. (TRUE)

3. Relapse is a natural part of the change process. (TRUE)

4. It is okay to hate yourself for relapsing as long as you start again. (FALSE)

5. The longer you maintain a new behavior, the more likely you are to relapse. (FALSE)

6. Personal lifestyle behaviors are personal so they only affect yourself. (FALSE)

7. World wellness recognizes an interconnectedness between ourselves and our environment. (TRUE)

8. During change, the human-cultural environment made up of the people closest to you is the most important. (TRUE)

9. Experiencing other human-cultural environments broadens your perspective and raises awareness. (TRUE)

10. Healthy lifestyle habits occasionally conflict with traditional beliefs. (TRUE)

11. Language and culture shape a person's thinking but have little influence over lifestyle choices. (FALSE)

12. Technology has, in some cases, added stress to people's lives. (TRUE)

13. A world view is human-centered. (FALSE)

14. A rooftop garden in the city is part of the natural environment. (TRUE)

15. There are very few things that one person can do to enhance the wellness of the natural environment. (FALSE)

Essay/Short Answer Questions

1. Describe three ways that we are insulated from the effects of the natural environment.

2. Give two positive and two negative examples of how:
   a. an individual affects the human-cultural environment
   b. an individual affects the natural environment
   c. the human-cultural environment affects the individual
   d. the natural environment affects the individual

3. Describe a situation in which one person's healthy lifestyle change makes another person uncomfortable.

4. Describe five ways you can experience an alternate human-cultural environment without leaving your state.

5. Identify five things you can do for the natural environment.